```
MW01538586
```

Many thanks for your
Kind help —

Sidney Ledson
(essel@bell.net)

Also by Sidney Ledson

Grammar for People Who Hate Grammar
Teach Your Child to Read in 60 Days
Raising Brighter Children
Teach Your Child to Read in Just Ten Minutes a Day
Give Your Child Genius IQ

Humor
Scratch 'n' Win

Under the pseudonym "Sister Trillium"
Talk About a Bad Hair Day!
Off My Skateboard, Granny

DON'T BOTHER
Living to 90
WITHOUT THIS BOOK

Sidney Ledson

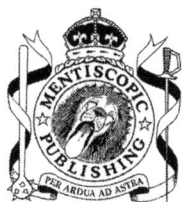

MENTISCOPIC PUBLISHING

PER ARDUA AD ASTRA

Copyright © 2016 by Sidney Ledson

All rights reserved. No part of this publication may be repro-
duced, stored in a retrieval system, or transmitted, in any
form or by any means, electronic, mechanical, photocopying,
recording or otherwise, without prior written permission of
the publisher or author. Contact essel@bell.net.

20 19 18 17 16 1 2 3 4 5

ISBN 978-1533392213

Cover design: Sidney Ledson

Contents

1
"Your Money or Your Life!"
An Attractive Deal

This life-insurance proposal, voiced by seventeenth-century highwaymen in England, left little room for haggling. (Sorry, my golden guineas are all in my other breeches.) Yet, strangely, it's a better deal than is offered today by cigarette manufacturers, burger merchants, and confectionary artists, who, while taking your money, will take your life as well. You don't believe it? Most people don't. And that's why so many wither and fall like fruit from the vine long before they reach the age of ninety.

But wait! Who wants to live to ninety anyway? The gag answer is: *Everyone who's eighty-nine.* For most people, though, the vision of a white-haired ninety-, eighty-, or even seventy-year-old shuffling along with a cane or bent over a walker — hampered further, perhaps, by muddled thinking — paints a gloomy picture of life's later years: an experience to be avoided if possible. But the elder years can be entirely different, and each of us has the power to help make them so. Activities you engage in today — or fail to — are already extending or limiting the abilities you will still have when you reach the later years. You are in the catbird seat. You call the shots. You dictate your future performance. What's your pleasure?

Reaching nine-zero is relatively unimportant. It's good health, vigor, mental acuity, and a sunny disposition that ring bells (which is true, of course, whether you're ninety or just fifty). And these desirable traits are malleable; they will wax or wane according to your prevailing thoughts and habits. This book shows you how to cash in on the best that life has to offer during your upcoming years. And believe me, there's plenty for you to enjoy.

But doesn't luck play a part?

You bet. And it already has. The fact that you are breathing today is because you haven't filled the starring role in a fatal car accident, stopped a bullet (intended, perhaps, for someone else), or succumbed to a lightning strike or a deadly disease or some other chance mortality. Luck has already played an important role in your present existence, and it will continue to do so.

What if your parents died long before they reached ninety? Doesn't that put a damper on your extended presence? This common belief isn't endorsed by research. The 20% to 30% programming acquired genetically at birth holds sway primarily during the early years. However, it diminishes as environmental forces gradually exert their influence, and disappears entirely in the later years.

Studies conducted at the University of Gothenburg show that lifestyle plays a far greater role in determining longevity than inherited genes. The report, published in the *Journal of Internal Medicine*, described 855 men born in 1913 who were examined at ages fifty, fifty-four, sixty, seventy-five, and eighty. The researchers found that the participants who didn't smoke, consumed just moderate amounts of coffee, and were still physically active at age fifty-four outlived the others regardless of their genes.

These findings are consistent with those from the Swedish Twin Registry study, which reported: "Among pairs ... in which both [twins] lived until very old age, the variance in age of death seemed to have no genetic component. Model fitting procedures [of twins] reared apart and twins reared together indicate that most of the variance in longevity was explained by environmental factors."

So the good news is you can reach ninety — and even older — in good health, sound of wind, and sharp of mind, if you sow the seeds today for that more active later life. The purpose of this book is to show you how to do so.

Nonagenarians aren't necessarily the best authorities on how to reach ninety. It's all very well to cite a glass of Scotch before bed or church attendance and prayer or the lavishing of olive oil on your food and skin (as some have), but these notions aren't supported by research (except, perhaps, by virtue of a possible placebo effect).

So what keeps me wound up and ticking? Nothing magical — just nutritious foods; a busy, active life; a fun-loving nature; and abundant interests, all of which, individually, have consistently been found to contribute to health and longevity. I weigh 128 pounds (58.6 kg), which, at a height of 5 feet, 7 inches (170 cm), produces a body mass index of 20 (raising the question at what point does "slim" devolve into "skinny"?). However, low weight doesn't necessarily indicate good health; one might be fragile or even ill. (If that light weight catches your eye, you may find the secret of comfortable weight management in Chapter 4 of value.)

I can't remember a time when I had a major illness. I take no medications (a matter discussed more fully in later chapters) and I'm usually mistaken for someone younger. I recently moved fifty heavy wheelbarrow-loads of material unaided and suffered no discomfort — hardly a gold-medal performance, admittedly. I hope to do better at jogging, to which I'm just returning (though I'm having a tough time getting beyond even a laughable 300 yards, so stay tuned).

Household chores help to keep me active, as do my three dogs, whose combined weight is 100 pounds more than my own. They make the game of home management more challenging by rearranging the furniture and carpets (canine feng shui) and coating everything with hair. Their two off-leash runs in a forested park each day provide two miles of walking for me, though I sometimes pamper myself with a brief fifteen- or twenty-minute nap following such outings, especially on hot days (snap-naps and how to enlist their restful value are covered in Chapter 7).

But these are just routine achievements, not newsworthy triumphs. Still, some older folks might find interesting biomarkers in them. I do have a few non-debilitating ailments and a touch of arthritis. Now, if the medical's over, I'll put my shirt back on.

You, the reader, may have more serious afflictions — perhaps heart problems, diabetes, or excess weight — and you may want to avoid becoming a burden to others when you're older. Or perhaps you have a loved one whose condition needs ongoing care and improvement. Dealing as we are with various matters pertaining to different ages and different stages of health, you may be prompted to jump around to find information specific to your needs. For that, you'll need to know what this book includes. Here is a chapter-by-chapter glance at the contents.

Chapter 2: Scaling Healthful Heights: "Move over, Ar-r-rnold!"

Possibly the most common benchmark by which advanced age is judged desirable or not is mobility. What can the elder still do? Pole-vaulting and tossing the caber are probably out, but what important daily tasks can he or she perform? Simple and easy ways to gradually improve movement and physical ability are revealed.

Chapter 3: How to Avoid the Hooks, Lures, and Perils at Your Supermarket

The moment you stroll into a supermarket, you are fingered as an impressionable mark, one to be inclined this way or that and induced to purchase specific chosen foods. Taste merchants await your approach with their eye-catching products. You are targeted. Look out!

Chapter 4: Free Tummy-Tuck Performed on Your Kitchen Table Without Anesthetic

You get it from all sides these days, don't you? *Don't eat junk food!* Yet sales remain brisk and their stocks earn favorable returns as manufacturers of these delicious edibles continue to churn out their health-destroying products, cheered on (chewed on?) by their countless salivating customers. We examine hair-raising details of this popular form of slow suicide and the astonishing power of the resultant gut flora problems it creates. Learn too how autosuggestion can make changes in eating habits easier to stomach (pun).

Chapter 5: Laugh Your Way to Health

Reader's Digest has said so for decades, and every study undertaken of the subject confirms their assertion. And yet, strangely enough, the exalted prize — a sense of humor — is rarely understood and seldom acquired. How to develop this skill for your personal enjoyment and harness its potential for health and social advantage are described.

Chapter 6: Hold Still, We're Working on Your Brain

Fitness buffs work frenetically at the gym to improve their physical performance, yet rarely think to similarly exercise their brain. Pity. "Use it or lose it" applies equally to muscles and to cerebral tissue. Easy ways to rev up your cranial motor are revealed.

Chapter 7: Why Hitchhike? Take the Bullet Train to Dreamland

Sufficient rest gives you the strength to slay your daily quota of mastodons or to deal with whatever other fearsome challenges you face. But sleep doesn't come easily to everyone, and though insufficient rest presents problems at any age, it exacts a steeper price for older people. Learn how to use self-hypnosis to put yourself to sleep quickly, either at night or for daytime snap-naps, and how, surprisingly, you can put your body to sleep, then open your eyes and carry on a conversation. Freaky? Maybe, but it's worth knowing.

Chapter 8: The Twenty-Four Vertebrae Blues

A hunched posture, common to older folks, isn't an affliction you have to accept passively. Simple everyday practices can inhibit and counter this unfortunate slumping habit.

Chapter 9: Company Comin' Up the Road — Get Out 27,000 Chairs

Long before you reach age ninety, vacancies start appearing in your circle of friends. Making new friends can be difficult or not, depending on how you go about it. Methods that have worked for others and will work for you are revealed.

Chapter 10: The World's Your Oyster, So Eat

It's difficult in just one lifetime to peruse and enjoy the countless delights arrayed about this engaging world of ours. But we can try. Fascinating activities that you might not have previously considered or allowed into your schedule — some with healthful surprises — are dealt with.

Chapter 11: Showbiz in the Home

How you act influences both your health and happiness, so if you've ever thought of acting, now's a good time to start. You'll find that life's pleasures become more bountiful for the price of a small dramatic performance each day. Immediate audition — no waiting.

Chapter 12: Welcome to Ninety

So you've hit ninety. What surprises can you expect and what treats will now be yours? It's a time for elation, not gloom.

2
Scaling Healthful Heights
"Move over, Ar-r-rnold!"

Those who think they have not time for bodily exercise
will sooner or later have to find time for illness.
— Edward Stanley, 15th Earl of Derby (1873)

Before 1960, the only adults you might see running were attempting to catch a bus or escaping something. And the only traffic moving in and out of gymnasiums was puffy-eyed pugilists and body-builders. The notion hadn't yet surfaced that muscular activity — exercise — could, or should, become a normal daily activity for everyone.

And there I've said it: the bothersome E-word that we now encounter on all sides. *Exercise*: a disruptive force that displaces more pleasing activities such as reading, watching TV, or just sitting in the garden dreamily studying cloud castles. Still, though we might wish otherwise, exercise holds the trump card where our health is concerned. Those who fail to include adequate physical activity in their lives pay a stiff price, ending in a fate from which I hope to spare you: frequent illnesses and a shortened lifespan.

CAUTION

If exercise could worsen an illness or affliction that you
are suffering, skip this chapter and begin with Chapter 3.

So here's this old fellow tapping away at a computer keyboard (and developing powerful sitting muscles) advising others how to boost their health by staying active. Guilty! But then I've reached ninety and you probably haven't. So hold your criticism, please, while I work out how we can get you into the nonagenarian fraternity or sorority.

Let's begin with the reason for all this fuss about staying active. The unpleasant truth — which I'm sure is neither new nor pleasing music to your ear — is that too much sitting is unhealthy. No, let's give it full orchestral amplification. Scientific studies prove that ***excessive sitting is a slow, comfortable, socially acceptable form of suicide***. Sorry, but it's a fact. Research shows, again and again, that the more time we spend applying butt to chair, the more we increase our risk of contracting diabetes, heart disease, and cancer — and, as a consequence, of course, shrinking our lifespan. (This sends a gloomy message to those whose job fastens them to a seat. Computer functionaries, commercial drivers, and [ahem] writers, take note.)

Exercise helps you maintain your present level of physical ability, and when you increase your exercise, you increase your muscular strength. That's how Arnold Schwarzenegger acquired his collection of balloon-sized muscles — and subsequent entry into the movies. (Hey, maybe we can get you into the movies too. Why not? They've never had a ninety-year-old Tarzan or Jane!)

Finally, evidence suggests that exercise helps prevent Alzheimer's disease. A study of seventy patients with mild cognitive impairment (which can lead to Alzheimer's) was conducted by Laura Baker of the Wake Forest School of Medicine. She found that those who engaged in supervised aerobics for forty-five minutes to an hour, four times a week, had a reduced level of tau, a protein associated with Alzheimer's. "These findings are important because they strongly suggest a potent lifestyle intervention such as aerobic exercise can impact Alzheimer's-related changes in the brain," Baker reported. "No currently approved medication can rival these effects."

Exercise provides a surprise service as an ever-present anesthetic, should you endure discomfort. When you exercise, your body releases chemicals called endorphins, which trigger a positive feeling similar to that produced by pain-relieving morphine — which is why the pleasant feeling that follows a run or a workout is often described as euphoric.

With potential winnings like these available to you in life's lottery, how many tickets would you like? That, friend, is what this book is all about:

helping you win a chance to leave the planet a lot later, and more pleasantly.

But first we need to consider your age. You might be anywhere from twenty to eighty, or even older. Let's assume you are between forty and fifty — say, forty-five. (Those who are younger or older can tailor their involvement in our pursuit of eternal youth accordingly.) Naturally, age will limit the physical activities you can wisely engage in and the degree of effort you should apply (which means no bronco-busting after seventy, and no kickboxing after eighty). Whatever your present capability, one thing is certain: you can increase your level of muscular activity at least a modest amount. Correct? That's all we need for the moment.

Fun and Games

Now for a surprise. What if I told you there's a playful activity — depicted, interestingly enough, in an Egyptian tomb dated 1781 BC — that provides a mind-boggling array of healthful advantages? This near game needs no expensive equipment, sharpens your focus, advances your concentration, relieves stress, improves both your hand-eye coordination and peripheral vision, and, to top it all off, increases your intelligence. The miracle activity? Juggling!

It's true. Studies show that every desirable attribute mentioned above is improved by the simple act of juggling. We'll get to the mechanical how-to of juggling in a moment. First we should consider that hard-to-believe claim of intellectual advancement.

Studies conducted at Oxford University's Department of Clinical Neurology show that juggling creates changes in the bundles of long fibers that conduct electrical signals between nerve cells. The scientists selected twenty-four healthy young adults, none of whom could juggle, divided them into two groups, and scanned their brains using diffusion magnetic resonance imaging (dMRI). One group then received weekly lessons in juggling and were asked to practice thirty minutes every day. The other twelve received no instruction or training. After just six weeks, MRI scans for the jugglers showed a 5% size increase in a rear section of their brain called the intraparietal sulcus.

The Oxford research team found that, while there was great variation in the ability of the volunteers to juggle, all of them generated neural growth. This made the team conclude that the important element of the exercise was the time spent practicing rather than the level of skill they achieved. Dr. Heidi Johansen-Berg, who led the study, said, "Knowing that pathways in the brain can be enhanced may be significant in the long run in coming up with new treatments for neurological diseases, such as multiple sclerosis, where these pathways become degraded."

So how do you begin? The Internet is fairly abuzz with sites eager to show you how to juggle. Several provide video demonstrations of the basic procedure. Your first step will be to buy a set of three juggling balls, available at sports stores or obtainable on the Internet. But while you're awaiting their delivery, I can get you started.

Create two balls by scrunching up sheets of newspaper or printer paper. Begin by holding a ball in each hand. Toss the ball in your right hand up, with the intention of catching it with your left hand. However, while the ball is in flight, throw the ball in your left hand sideways into your now-empty right hand. Continue with that procedure until you gain skill (it's tricky).

How long will it take to master this move? That depends on how much time you spend trying. But remember: the greater benefit — as documented by the research team at Oxford — lies not in advancing your juggling skill but in merely engaging in the exercise. You could become an Einstein and still be picking up balls from the floor. (Incidentally, you'll find that the major exercise component comes from picking up missed balls.)

When you've developed facility with the routine, reverse the procedure described above. Toss up the ball in your left hand with the intention of catching it in your right hand. While it's in transit, transfer the ball in your right hand sideways into your now-empty left hand.

In time you can attempt to juggle three balls. The procedure is more easily understood if you watch the demonstrations on the Internet. When I began juggling with three balls, it was a big event when I caught them five times in a row. Gradually I was able to get up to ten balls, then continued on to higher numbers, reaching a peak in the sixties. However, my usual count during a five-minute daily practice is between twenty and thirty.

Getting started with juggling takes courage. Like everything you attempt for the first time, it can seem difficult. But concentrate on the several rewards that competency provides. Oh, and when you're with an unsuspecting friend or associate, you'll be able to say, "Excuse me a moment, the iridium plates in my shoulders are itching again." Produce three balls, juggle a quick ten-count, and then put the balls away. "Yes, that's better. Now, you were saying . . . ?" Or, if you're really confident, when you're in the produce department at the supermarket, pick up three oranges and dazzle the attendant.

Just reading these words isn't enough. You have to tackle the challenge with resolve. When I heard that an acquaintance would be losing her driving license because her peripheral vision was failing, I explained the proven value of juggling to remedy that weakness. Her response? She can't juggle. *Of course she can't juggle. She's never tried it.* Don't let the four-letter, failure-prone word *can't* defeat you before you try.

Riding Shank's Mare

In decades past, walking was the way people commonly moved around. It wasn't unusual for walkers to journey ten, fifteen, or twenty miles in a half-day. The practice has greatly diminished since automobiles arrived, and this, regrettably, has adversely influenced public health. It's time to resurrect the activity for your benefit, which is of infinitely greater importance as you age.

Studies conducted at the University of Iowa show that differences in brain health in older adults vary with physical fitness levels. The researchers reported: "Our study provides the strongest evidence to date that fitness in an older adult population can have substantial benefits to brain health in terms of the functional connections of different regions of the brain." Physical fitness among the elderly provides stronger brain connections and improves long-term brain function.

These findings were echoed by researchers at King's College London after studying 324 healthy female twins over a ten-year period, beginning in 1999. Thinking, learning, and memory were measured at both the beginning and end of the study. Scientists learned that leg power was a better predictor of cognitive change than any other lifestyle factor tested. Generally the twin who had more leg power at the start of the study sustained her cognition better and had fewer brain changes associated with aging after ten years.

Walking is an activity that lends itself to easy incremental advancement. Pick up a fitness tracker from any of the sources listed on the Internet and keep track of the number of steps you walk in a day.

Keep track of the total steps walked during a three-
or four-day period, then divide the total by the
number of days to learn the average number taken
each day. With this figure you can plan a program
of gradual daily advancement.

Here you have a choice of how quickly you want
to progress. If, for example, you choose to walk just
ten steps more each day than you did the previous
day, at the end of a year you'll be walking an additional 3,650 steps daily — roughly 1.25 miles (2 km).
Not bad! And remember, this amount is *in addition
to* the routine daily distance you were walking before you began your advancement program. Still,
you may find — as others have — that you begin to
challenge your former unmotivated self and try to
advance more quickly. If so, good. The more time
and effort you put into advancing your health, the
better.

You might prefer a different procedure, perhaps
walking a hundred steps each day for a week or
two, then adding a hundred steps, and continuing
on in this way, adding weekly increments of a hundred steps. Whichever procedure you favor and the
degree of effort you decide to give it are of less importance than the fact that you actually get started
with your pursuit of health.

A treadmill permits you to walk anytime you
wish — of particular value when it's raining or
snowing. But when the sun is shining and the birds
are singing, outdoor walking is far healthier for you,
according to studies conducted at the University of

Essex. Researchers found that just a small dose of nature — only five minutes each day — benefits your mood, self-esteem, and mental health. It seems that flowers, trees, birds, and bees have an unsuspected secret role to play in our lives.

Now, erupting like a black cloud from these thoughts I've been weaving, is the depressing word *bother*. The program is a bother. Yes, it is, admittedly. But it's a more pleasant bother than being wheeled feet first from your dwelling by paramedics. Changing a familiar, comfortable routine is undeniably inconvenient, even unpleasant. And there's always the greater attraction of doing nothing. An easy, relaxing lifestyle needs no slick ad campaign to attract millions of eager participants.

I know the lure. I'm as guilty as anyone. Sometimes when I'm out walking the dogs, I think how nice it would be to ride in a vehicle like the one in which Alec Guinness floated along just above the ground in *Star Wars*. So when motivation is flagging, top up your enthusiasm by reflecting on CODA ("the end") — Cancer, Obesity, Diabetes, and Alzheimer's. And let's paste a recognizable, suitably threatening face onto those words before we assess what danger they hold for you.

Roughly thirty million North Americans are afflicted by diabetes and ninety million have prediabetes, which means their blood sugar is too high and they will likely become full-blown diabetics within ten years. That's strike one.

Weight? Reportedly one in three junk food–munchers is obese, while two out of three are merely overweight. Look around you for proof. Strike two!

Continuing our dreary trek through the medical reports, we learn there are more than a hundred different types of cancer, and this arsenal of deadly spikes will eliminate one in four of us. Foul ball! You get another chance.

Finally, nearly forty-four million people world-wide have Alzheimer's or a related dementia. *Pop!* — a fly ball.

Now what percentage of the population isn't getting enough exercise? Well, we're not really concerned about the general population here. We're interested in just one person — *you*. So slide into first base. Safe!

If you spend your day in an office, ways to exercise are limited. At one time when I worked in a high-rise, I'd take the elevator down ten stories, then climb back up via the stairs. Try it. Start with just three or four floors and gradually increase the challenge. Do you live in a high-rise? If so, try getting off the elevator a few floors short of your apartment and climb the rest of the way.

You may be attracted to a more aggressive program of healthy advancement. If so, consider jogging (almost a neighborhood sport these days). I'm not suggesting that you jog a mile or two. I mean just fifty strides or paces — a small amount you can gradually increase by five or ten paces a day, pursuing the easy progression suggested for walking. Your nature and your circumstances will largely determine how quickly you begin your program and whether it's to be walking or jogging. There are other simple ways to increase your mobility. For example, when you visit the supermarket, park your car in the slot farthest from the store. Or, indeed, how about walking to the supermarket with your own buggy? Did someone say "ouch"?

Strangely, the invention of the wheel, a major technological advancement, has often exacted a penalty in health. Grace Halsell, who studied the elders of Vilcabamba in the mountains of Ecuador, where eighty- and ninety-year-olds enjoy top fitness and health, says, "They've never been handicapped by the wheel as a mode of transport. They own no cars nor bicycles. They simply walk." There's a saying in Vilcabamba that each of us has two doctors: the left leg and the right leg.

The immediate excuse for avoiding energy-tapping tasks is that you haven't time. This equates, alas, to not having time to be healthy, which (in one further nonsensical step) means you haven't time to stay alive. This sort of thinking will get the undertaker busy polishing an elaborate mahogany overcoat for you. Don't forget, I'm on your side. I want to keep you out of the pre-burial cosmetician's hands. Despite his services and art, you look nicer alive.

You know better that anyone how urgently you need to escape a way of life that at the moment is promising neither health nor longevity. So map out a program of proposed activities for yourself. That's the first step. Having done so, you need to be sure that you will honor your commitment to those activities every day. With other pressing matters on your mind, it's all too easy to forget. The solution? Coming right up.

The Daily Reminder

One way to make forgetting difficult is to create a grid listing the days of the month down one side and your planned activities across the top. Keep the grid where you can't avoid seeing it during the day (the kitchen counter, perhaps) and tick off the appropriate box as you execute each activity.

I've now suggested various approaches that will help you begin a healthful advancement at whatever gentle pace you find comfortable. The important point, however, is that you actually get started. Perhaps you're still in a "maybe" stage, sitting, as it were, on the end of a diving board and wondering whether you should jump in or wait for a friendly push. If so, may I offer a suggestion fresh from our Friendly Push Department.

Autosuggestion

Autosuggestion, a cousin of autohypnosis, is a power you've probably already used at various times without realizing it. The procedure, which I use occasionally, can help you overcome any reluctance you might have about performing the activities entered on your exercise grid. Here's the procedure.

Consider first the power of a simple suggestion. Suppose you're dining with a friend at a seafood restaurant. While you're studying the menu, your friend says, "The baked clams here are delicious. Why don't you try them?" This artless suggestion is likely to influence your choice of food (unless, of course, you don't like clams). Autosuggestion works similarly, except it's a suggestion you make to yourself. Strangely, it can actually bend your thoughts and actions.

Suppose, for example, you're reluctant to try the unattractive practice mentioned earlier, of parking your car a distance from your proposed destination and then walking the rest of the way. Make the suggestion to yourself in a roundabout way, thinking, *I wonder what it would be like to park the car a block from [location] and walk the rest of the way. Probably wouldn't kill me. [Name of person] would laugh when I told [him/her] what I'd done. Might try it. Hey, perhaps I'd lose an ounce or two, or even enough to register on the scale.* At this point, turn your thoughts to some other matter. It's best if you forget what you've just considered. By forgetting the suggestion you allow your subconscious to take control.

Later, when you actually make your visit to the place in question, you might find that a pleasant notion invades your thinking. It suggests that you try, "just this once," parking the car short of your destination and walking the rest of the way. When you've done so, be sure to congratulate yourself on this great success. *Well, that wasn't too painful. Might try it again sometime.* That's the way a healthy habit can start.

One powerful form of suggestion has attracted much medical attention: the placebo effect. You probably know that just to believe in the healing power of some nostrum will sometimes produce a cure even though the "medication" actually has no healing ability. More astonishing still, studies have shown that even when patients are told in advance that the pill they have been given has no healing properties, it still diminishes their nagging symptoms.

This mysterious power generates sales of copper bracelets to ease arthritic pain and various other maladies. Quack medicine? Of course it is, but it reduces pain for approximately 30% of the population. For them the curative power is real and they don't mind being laughed at. An older friend of mine, a medical doctor, used to wear a twisted copper wire around his wrist, and he vouched for its effectiveness in reducing his discomfort.

Tobacco Road

I see someone at the back lighting up a cigarette, so we'd best stop and discuss the problem. Nonsmokers can skip the following text.

First, the good news. A study shows that smokers who exercise live as long as, or even longer than, nonsmokers who don't exercise. We've all heard how bad smoking is, but to avoid exercise is apparently even worse. And that, I regret, ends the good news. It's all downhill from here.

I smoked for twenty-nine years, so kicking the habit is a task I've experienced. Some claim that nicotine is the addictive force. I don't believe it. The addiction is one of habit.

Consider the force of habit. Circumstances recently obliged me to begin wearing my watch on my right wrist instead of my left. The change wasn't difficult so long as I thought about the change while putting on the watch. If I had some other matter on my mind, the device invariably ended up on the wrong wrist — and this error persisted for months. Now compare the breaking of this habit to what is faced in breaking the habit of smoking.

During, say, a ten-year period I had placed the watch on my left wrist 3,650 times (365 days × 10 years). However, during the same ten-year period I would have smoked twenty cigarettes a day. That's 10 × 20 × 365 = 73,000 cigarettes, generating a force to continue smoking that was twenty times stronger than my choice of which wrist to wear my watch on.

Understandably, smokers become canny about finding justification for continuing their habit, pointing out, for example, that some ninety-year-olds have smoked all their lives and seemingly suffered no harm. They have indeed, and some people have won the lottery. But counting on lottery-type odds to keep you out of a casket isn't a wise bet. Over the years I've heard many quaint reasons to avoid quitting. One is "I can quit smoking anytime I want. I just don't want to." Here's another: "Giving up smoking's easy. I've done it several times."

Nicotine patches, anyone? Patches might work for roughly 30% of the population, but it's because of their placebo effect, not their nicotine content. Smokers expect the patch to diminish their urge to smoke — and so it does. They have inadvertently employed autosuggestion (there's more on autosuggestion in Chapter 4, by the way). Studies show e-cigarettes to be as effective as nicotine patches, which seems to suggest that we're just playing games with placebo expectations.

There are also spurious ways to supposedly make quitting easier. One is to gradually cut back on the number of cigarettes you smoke each day. This works only until pressing business or family matters take over your thoughts; then it's back to "normal" smoking. Another ruse is to make cigarettes difficult to obtain by keeping them on another floor, thereby requiring an annoying trip for each cigarette. But you soon learn that you will travel to any point short of the moon to satisfy your demand for a smoke.

I tried these false methods but finally escaped the habit in the only way that works: cold turkey. And yet even today, almost fifty years later, I sometimes find myself smoking in a dream. Suddenly realizing what I'm doing, all I can say is, "I thought I gave this up!"

The Four-Legged, Tail-Wagging Health Provider

Dogs coax you to exercise, even when you'd rather rest. My three promptly remind me when it's time for a run, and though the lure of a chair and interesting reading matter is always present, conscience kills choice, and we're out the door for another healthful trek. We live near a wooded park that abounds with wildlife, including deer, coyotes, foxes, raccoons, and rabbits. There my three can run off-leash, so, while I practice singing (more on that later), they coach squirrels in climbing trees faster.

All right, you're bustin' to know about my dogs, right? Front and center there's Robin, age thirteen, half German shepherd, half border collie. Emerging from the wings there's Spence, age six, a purebred border collie (a strange, one-person dog). And towering over the medium-sized dogs is young Kim, age three, a hundred-pound long-haired German shepherd.

Pet ownership has awakened surprising interest and applications in the fields of commerce and medicine. For example, older applicants for life insurance at the Midland Life Insurance Company of Columbus, Ohio, become eligible for a more favorable rate if they have a pet. And children who share the company of dogs are found to be less likely to develop allergies or asthma. Research shows that heart patients survive longer if they have a dog or cat. In one study, stockbrokers with high blood pressure who adopted a cat or dog were found to have lower blood pressure readings in stressful situations than did people without pets. Playing with a dog has been seen to elevate levels of serotonin and dopamine, nerve transmitters that deliver a pleasant calming sensation (the same high that users of heroin and cocaine seek). People with AIDS reportedly suffer less depression if they have a pet.

Ownership of a pet has also been found to provide power against the silent killer, stress. Stress generates production of cortisol and norepinephrine, chemicals that depress the immune system — which virtually puts out a welcome mat for any passing infection. These same chemicals build plaque in the arteries, which of course promotes heart disease. In 1980 a clinical research project at Brooklyn College, New York, studied heart-disease patients after their discharge from the hospital. Researchers tracked each survivor, studying their medical histories, lifestyles, families, and relationships. They reported: "The presence of a pet was the strongest social predictor of survival — not just for lonely or depressed people, but everyone — independent of marital status and access to social support from human beings." Another report found that ownership of pets lowered visits to the doctor by 21%.

And now, lest any of us get carried away by our seemingly impressive physical abilities, let's consider a real champion.

Jack Lalanne

I believe the world owes Jack Lalanne a standing ovation for showing us what the human body — yours and mine — can do when given appropriate nourishment and exercise. Consider his conquests. To prove it was possible to escape from Alcatraz, the maximum-security US penal center, Lalanne swam from Alcatraz Island to Fisherman's Wharf, San Francisco — a distance of about a mile — while wearing handcuffs. At age forty-five he completed 1,000 push-ups and 1,000 chin-ups in an hour and twenty-two minutes. At sixty he again swam from Alcatraz to Fisherman's Wharf while both hand-cuffed and shackled, this time towing a 1,000-pound boat. And at seventy, handcuffed, shackled, and battling currents, he towed seventy boats holding seventy people for a mile and a half across Long Beach Harbor. (Some of us might want to sit down and rest for a few minutes before we tackle that, even without the passengers.)

But wait — his accomplishments don't end there. He also advocated body-building exercise for women and weightlifting for older folks, at a time when doctors predicted disastrous injuries for both.

We might naturally assume that, given an appropriate early start with the correct foods and with exercise and guidance, some of us might have accomplished as much. But Jack Lalanne lacked all three. As a teenager, he had to drop out of school for a year because he was so ill. Thin, weak, and sickly, he had pimples and boils and wore a back brace. "I also had blinding headaches every day," he recalled. "I wanted to escape my body because I could hardly stand the pain. My life appeared hopeless." On learning that Lalanne was eating cake, pie, and ice cream for breakfast, lunch, and dinner, pioneer nutritionist Paul Bragg chastised the lad and inspired him to begin eating healthy foods.

Think of it, at age fourteen, you and I were miles ahead of Lalanne. We were strong and healthy, while he wasn't well enough to attend school. But now, ah, we have a little catching up to do. How to start?

The Gymnasium Alternative

You might think that visits to a commercial gym will suit your purpose. If that works for you, fine. But studies show that 67% of those who join a gym don't go there, and an even greater number fail to attend regularly. According to a 2005 study, gym attendance for most members is lower than 4.8 times per month. Even that little is certainly better than none at all, but occasional exercise isn't what we're aiming for here. However, there is one readily available source of exercise, and though it doesn't build bulging muscles, it nevertheless helps keep us active and limber.

I live in a small bungalow. As you perhaps know, no matter which point of the compass you face in a house, there is something to be cleaned, put away, repaired, dusted, replaced, painted, or tossed out. Then there are leaves to rake, the garden to weed, eavestroughs to clean, screens to vacuum, and other tasks that constantly demand attention. In short, to keep a house from looking abandoned and marginally above a state of squalor, you are kept in constant motion, despite your wishes.

At one time I made the mistake of hiring others to take care of various household chores, until it dawned on me that I was paying other people to stay healthy. I was operating what was virtually a private healthcare clinic — and paying the clientele to engage in health-promoting activities!

A house is a gym of sorts, with an endless program of necessary activities that drive old folks into the welcoming shelter of retirement homes — a comfortable path to a shorter life. As studies repeatedly show, it is constant activity that favors a long, healthy, energetic life. (Though sometimes — say, when kneeling on the bathroom floor cleaning around the toilet — I find that this promise of favor has limp appeal.)

Any group or tribe that enjoys longevity invariably endures a physically demanding existence. Many are farmers. The food they eat also has a major contributory influence to staying healthy and young in spirit. It's similar to the diet prescribed by Jack Lalanne, a matter discussed in the next chapter.

3
How to Avoid the Hooks, Lures, and Perils at Your Supermarket

This chapter is not about losing weight. Nor is it about dieting. It's about strengthening your body's ability to combat bacteria and viruses and helping keep you alive and healthy. It's about your immune system and the vital role food plays in maintaining its power.

In any discussion of food, confusion easily arises when it comes to distinguishing between nourishing foodstuffs and what are merely edibles. Worse, there's no clear line between the two. Some edibles are more nutritious than others, so we have to cautiously choose those foods that will produce the results we want.

You like puzzles? All right, here's a puzzle. Who do you suppose has made the greatest lasting impact on modern world cuisine? A French chef, Escoffier perhaps? Or Point, or Brazier? No, sorry, it was E.C. Segar. Hold it, E.C. *who*? Well might you ask. Though his name is forgotten, Segar, an American cartoonist, unintentionally changed eating habits in every English-speaking nation (and a few others) when he gave birth to a one-eyed, pipe-smoking sailor named Popeye in his popular newspaper comic strip, *Thimble Theater*. During the 1930s,

Popeye led youngsters (including me) to eat spinach and, what's more, to like it.

But Popeye never achieved the explosive food-related acceptance won by another character in the same comic strip: J. Wellington Wimpy, a rotund gentleman who encouraged readers to share his love of hamburgers. The simple meat patty sandwiched in a bun of Wimpy's cartoon day has expanded in girth and grandeur. The addition of mustard, cheese, onion, bacon, lettuce, tomato, dill pickle, and relish has turned it into an epic, mouth-watering work of art culminating in the Big Mac, which has twice as much of almost everything that could send you to an earlier grave. (And though E.C. Segar is gone, Wimpy lives on in a British chain of fast-food restaurants bearing his name. The specialty of the house is — guess what!)

At baseball arenas, big sales of another gastronomical hazard — the hotdog — have declined, along with ballpark attendance. (Do you suppose the hotdogs helped to kill off the fans?) Whereas the French gave Americans the Statue of Liberty, the Germans gave Americans the hotdog. German sausages and rolls were sold as "dachshund sandwiches" to fans at the old New York Polo Grounds in the 1890s. A *New York Post* cartoonist couldn't spell *dachshund*, so when he drew a cartoon about them, he called them "hot dogs."

And the Italians' donation? Ah yes, pizza.

Today hamburgers, hotdogs, and pizza are considered acceptable foods. They have nutritional value, yes, but their limited nutrients come with a heavy caloric overload, and foods with an unfavorable imbalance between nutrition and calories are what obesity is all about. That's the secret. That's why extra weight and obesity are common — not because people are eating too much but because the foods they eat have too many calories. Does that mean you can eat all the food you want, so long as it's the right type? Correct. That's largely the reason why I'm able to shovel in more food than I should and still weigh less than 130 pounds.

Obesity tends to run in families, and there's often an unsuspected reason. The poor eating habits that create heavy parents can work mightily to influence their heavy offspring's food preferences. But surprisingly, many overweight people are actually undernourished. Proof? It's seen when their immune system performs too ineffectively to fight off bacterial, parasitic, fungal, and viral infections, obliging the afflicted to endure frequent fatigue, allergies, colds, and flu.

If you rarely eat hot-off-the-griddle hamburgers, hot dogs, or pizza, good for you. However, you don't have to visit fast-food eateries anymore to find high-calorie edibles that are low in nutrients. The shelves of your supermarket are crowded with mouth-watering preparations heavily laden with salt, sugar, or fat — sometimes all three — and usually containing so many additives and fillers that only a chemistry major can be certain what is being sent down to the stomach. By eating what everyone else eats, consumers can easily form the idea that they are benefiting from the "safety in numbers" factor. Of course, they aren't, which is why few people reach age ninety, and those few are often in a pitiable condition.

The standard American diet — revolving as it does around meat, high in saturated fats, low in plant-based foods and complex carbohydrates — has prompted the Centers for Disease Control and Prevention to report that 39.5% of adults 40 to 59 years old are obese. Of younger adults, aged 20 to 39, 30.3% are obese, and 35.4% of adults over 60. Excess weight induces weight-related ailments, which include heart disease, stroke, and diabetes. Cardiovascular disease — the leading cause of death in North America — is less prevalent in vegetarians than in non-vegetarians. Vegetarians eat less animal fat and cholesterol (vegans consume none at all) and instead consume more fiber and more antioxidant-rich produce.

Dr. Michael F. Roizen, author of *The Real Age Diet: Make Yourself Younger with What You Eat*, claims that switching to a vegetarian diet can add about thirteen healthy years to your life. "People who consume saturated, four-legged fat have a shorter life span and more disability at the end of their lives. Animal products clog your arteries, zap your energy and slow down your immune system. Meat eaters also experience accelerated cognitive and sexual dysfunction at a younger age." Dr. Roizen's statements are based on countless reports and research studies that confirm the veracity and accuracy of his claims. We ignore his findings at our peril.

If I've presented the supper table as a sort of war zone with numerous shell craters to nimbly avoid, I've done it with your good health in mind. You get only one life, and that's it. So reap all the benefits you can from that one life. With wise decisions about the food you eat, not only will you live longer, you'll be able to enjoy more fully the best that life has to offer during those extended years.

We all tend to overeat. Me too. A solution? Studies show that if we chew our food well and avoid watching TV or reading while eating, we will reduce the quantity of food we eat. Slower food consumption gives the brain time to register satiety, which occurs about twenty minutes after the last swallow. So, when you're eating, concentrate on the food. You'll enjoy it more too.

To my astonishment, I find that there are people who still eat white bread; this, decades after the initial reports of its low nutritional value. In his book *Healthy at 100*, which compares foods eaten by Earth's oldest living residents against those of the industrialized world, John Robbins says: "Do you know why they call it Wonder Bread? Because if you eat it, it's a wonder you're still alive."

I don't know if you have any interest in knowing what I eat, but I'll list the components for you, to scan or to skip.

How to Eat Your Way to Health

My meals are simple, one might even say primitive. Breakfast is the same every morning:

- rolled oats and ground flax seeds (premixed half-and-half and stored in quantity)
- ground cinnamon
- raisins and blueberries (both washed, soaked, and kept in quantity in the fridge)
- canned peaches (well rinsed to eliminate the syrup)
- prunes (washed in quantity, boiled lightly, and stored)
- pumpkin seeds and sunflower seeds (ground and mixed half-and-half)
- an orange or kiwifruit (sometimes both)

Preparation is easy despite the many items, because all the components are quick to add after the oat-and-flaxseed mixture has boiled. Grape juice or unsweetened applesauce adds moisture to the mix. It's a non-fattening meal and you can eat as much as you want. Of note: each component contributes valuable health-promoting power, the antioxidants being possibly the most important.

Antioxidants are compounds that protect cells from damage caused by free radicals, which are unstable molecules that result from normal cell metabolism, smoking, pollution, and ultraviolet irradiation. Research suggests that free radicals may contribute to premature aging, wrinkling of the skin, cardiovascular disease, and certain types of cancer.

It isn't enough to say that my breakfast foods are merely healthful. Each makes an impressive nutritional contribution to the meal. Here they are:

- **Oats** are an excellent source of thiamine (vitamin B_1), iron, and dietary fiber, and are the only source of antioxidant compounds known as avenanthramides, which are believed to protect the circulatory system from arteriosclerosis.

- **Flax seeds** are a rich source of manganese, thiamine, omega-3 fatty acids, and dietary fiber. Flax seeds (and sesame seeds) contain more cancer-fighting lignans than any other foods. Their mucilage also lubricates and eases bowel movements.

- **Cinnamon** is high in cinnamaldehyde, which is responsible for its anti-inflammatory power. Containing large amounts of potent polyphenol antioxidants, cinnamon is also credited with reducing risk factors for high blood pressure and heart disease.

- **Raisins** are packed with several health-benefiting nutrients. Like fresh grapes, raisins contain the phytochemical compound resveratrol, a polyphenol antioxidant with anti-inflammatory power that generates blood cholesterol-lowering activities. Studies suggest that resveratrol affords protection against melanoma, colon and prostate cancer, coronary heart disease, degenerative nerve disease, Alzheimer's disease, and viral or fungal infections.

- **Blueberries**, whether wild or cultivated, are among the foods that contain the highest anti-oxidant capacity.
- **Canned peaches** come with a surprise. Studies show that canned peaches have higher levels of vitamin C, folate, and antioxidants than fresh peaches.
- **Prunes**, which have a long history of relieving constipation, have twice the antioxidant capacity of blueberries, topping even that of fresh plums. A study conducted at Florida State University found that dried plums reversed osteoporosis in postmenopausal women. Women who ate 100 grams of dried plums every day had improved bone formation–markers after only three months, compared to a control group that ate 75 grams of dried apples.
- **Pumpkin seeds** contain many health-benefiting vitamins, antioxidants, and essential amino acids and provide an impressive dose of minerals to the body. Research suggests that pumpkin seeds also cut the risk of prostate and ovarian cancers.
- **Sunflower seeds** contain thiamine, vitamin B_6, magnesium, phosphorus, copper, manganese, and selenium. They are also a rich source of vitamin E, which fights free radical damage in the body.

My lunch varies. Perhaps I'll spread some salt-free crushed tomatoes over a whole-wheat tortilla, then add romaine lettuce or some other vegetable.

Simple. The more I learn about nutrition, the more I've come to realize that the stomach is really a chemistry lab. The person "upstairs" might be interested in the appearance of food, its taste, smell, and texture, but when the chewed and mashed conglomerate travels down the esophagus, it mutates into a chemical assignment for the digestive system, whose job it is to sort out the nutrients and dispatch phytonutrients to their appropriate destinations.

Supper, a major production, is prepared thirty portions at a time, then frozen, so each meal requires only defrosting and warming of the components. Portobello or white button mushrooms are sliced and steam-cooked, as are garlic cloves, then distributed into Pyrex containers. These are the only vegetables to be cooked. All the others remain raw. Two red onions, two red bell peppers, and three heads of romaine lettuce are sliced and similarly distributed. Raisins, walnut pieces, blueberries, tofu, and a single sardine or small portion of wild (not farmed) salmon are added. Next, ground turmeric and black pepper are sprinkled on top, followed by olive oil, balsamic vinegar, and a dollop of unsweetened applesauce. The mixture receives a liberal squirt of horseradish sauce and is topped with a wafer of seaweed (for iodine).

Other foods occasionally included are broccoli, cauliflower, and Brussels sprouts, which, like all cruciferous vegetables, should be cooked before eating to protect the thyroid gland. Then there's canned spinach (rinsed free of salt) and green peas.

Some vegetables lend themselves to sprouting. Broccoli seeds (obtainable from garden suppliers) are easy to sprout. Studies at Johns Hopkins University have revealed that three- to four-day-old broccoli sprouts contain as much as fifty times the amount of certain health-boosting phytonutrients found in the mature broccoli head. The nutrient that makes broccoli sprouts exemplary is sulphoraphane, a compound with purported anticancer and anti-diabetic properties. Bean sprouts must be cooked to kill the bacteria they commonly harbor.

The entire preparation of thirty suppers, including cleanup, takes three hours, or six minutes each — remarkably quick for a meal containing so many components. Combining certain foods is believed to generate a synergistic phytonutrient power that exceeds the sum of their individual ingredients.

Exhaustive research prompted Dr. Joel Fuhrman, in his book *Eat to Live*, to rate greens, onions, mushrooms, and beans as superfoods. The exceptional health-promoting powers these foods contain might tempt you to include one or more of them in your own meals. So here they are:

Mushrooms give a mighty boost to the body's immune system, which declines as we age. The powerful nutritional content of these fungi (often wrongly thought of as vegetables) is enhanced when they are served with onions and green vegetables. Mushrooms, one of the few foods rich in vitamin D, contain phytochemicals that inhibit the growth of abnormal cells, tumors, and cancer. They are high in potassium and low in sodium, and thus help to lower blood pressure and decrease the risk of cardiovascular diseases. However, all mushrooms (even the edible type) contain toxins that are destroyed only by cooking, and some nutrients in the skin of mushrooms aren't released until they are cooked. Store mushrooms in a paper bag, not plastic — too much moisture hastens spoilage. And before eating, leave them in the sun for a while to increase their vitamin D content.

Garlic has been found to halve the risk of developing lung cancer. Researchers from the Jiangsu Provincial Center for Disease Control and Prevention in China collected data from 1,424 lung cancer patients alongside 4,543 healthy controls. Results showed that participants who consumed raw garlic two or more times a week had a 44% decrease in their risk of developing lung cancer. If you cook garlic, let it sit for a while between crushing and cooking, to increase its healthful power.

Onions contain anticancer, anti-inflammatory, and antioxidant compounds. A research study showed that a group of people who consumed a half-cup of chopped onions per day had a 56% reduction in colon cancer incidence, 73% reduction in ovarian cancer, 88% reduction in esophageal cancer, 71%

reduction in prostate cancer, and 50% reduction in stomach cancer.

Bell peppers are an excellent source of vitamins A and C, potassium, folic acid, and fiber. Red peppers are just green peppers that have stayed on the vine longer, which gives them a higher nutritional value. Compared to green peppers, the red variety contains almost eleven times more beta-carotene and 1.5 times more vitamin C. Before eating, remove wax from the skins of peppers by washing with a vegetable rinse (easily made by diluting vinegar or lemon juice with water and storing it in a spray bottle).

Romaine lettuce — truly a wonder food — is low in saturated fat and sodium and very low in cholesterol. It is also rich in riboflavin (vitamin B_2), calcium, magnesium, phosphorus, and copper. It is a good source of dietary fiber, vitamins A, B_6, C, and K, thiamine, folate, iron, potassium, and manganese.

Walnuts, like flax seeds, contain omega-3 fats, which balance out the damaging influence of the omega-6 fats common to North American diets. (Omega-6 fats increase the risk of heart disease, diabetes, and inflammatory illnesses such as rheumatoid arthritis and Crohn's disease.) A diet rich in omega-3s helps reduce depression, attention-deficit hyperactivity disorder, cancer, and Alzheimer's disease.

Tofu, an exceptional food, contains eight essential amino acids and a long list of health-promoting vitamins and minerals. Tofu is thought to provide the same sort of protection against cancer and heart disease as the soybeans from which it is made.

Sardines sit (or rather swim) near the bottom of the watery food chain and contain, in consequence, little of the mercury common to larger fish. Rich in niacin (vitamin B$_3$) and calcium, sardines are an excellent source of protein, vitamin D, vitamin B$_{12}$, phosphorus, and selenium.

Turmeric contains curcumin, which is responsible for the yellow color of Indian curry powder and American mustard. Curcumin has powerful antioxidant properties. Elderly villagers in India who eat turmeric with almost every meal have the lowest rate of Alzheimer's disease in the world. The curcumin in turmeric isn't well absorbed unless it is eaten with black pepper.

Peanut butter is a superfood that contains vitamin E, bone-building magnesium, muscle-friendly potassium, and immunity-boosting vitamin B$_6$. Research shows that eating peanuts decreases the risk of several chronic health conditions.

My usual dessert, though simple, provides a sweet enough ending to supper. It's always the same: a combination of unsweetened applesauce, processed high-fiber bran, raisins (washed and soaked), peach slices, peanut butter (unsalted), and grape juice. Mix these together in whatever proportions suit your taste and you get a delicious and healthy masterpiece. It's unexciting to look at, yes, but unlike store-bought cakes and pies, it contains no fillers, emulsifiers, coloring, flavor enhancers, or artificial sweeteners. So there you have it — plain and drab, yes, but nutritious and tasty.

A study of 100,000 people spanning three decades, published in the *New England Journal of Medicine*, found that people who ate nuts daily were 20% less likely to die over the thirty-year period, 29% less likely to suffer heart disease, and 11% less likely to die from cancer. Accordingly, a mixture of peanuts, Brazil nuts, walnuts, and cashews provides a powerful 2-ounce (60 g) burst of vitality for me every day.

Beverages include water, tea, coffee — caffeine, being a drug and not a food, is limited to one cup a day — grape juice (which contains resveratrol), and an unsalted mixed-vegetable drink. A word might be in order about coffee, which provides a surprising unexpected health benefit. The *Journal of the American Medical Association* described a thirty-year follow-up study of 8,004 men aged 45 to 68 that showed coffee drinkers had a lower risk of Parkinson's disease (PD). The relationship between caffeine and PD was unaltered by intake of milk and sugar.

Wine, beer, whisky, vodka — what's your choice? Alcohol has filled variously important parts in my life, but it doesn't now. Oh, I might consume one small glass of organic wine before supper, but wine drinkers will be nonplussed to learn that the glass often holds an equal quantity of grape juice.

My supplements include vitamin D_3 (1,000 IU), which is advised for older people, especially those who, like me, live in "northern latitudes." (Since I live in Toronto, this will prompt residents of the Northwest Territories to snort, slap their thighs, and howl with teary-eyed laughter.) Zinc (50 mg) fills several vital roles in maintaining health. Because the body can't store zinc for future use, it must be ingested daily.

Omega-3 fatty acids, ingested periodically, are seen to benefit cardiovascular health, so occasionally I take fish oil capsules (500 mg). An Italian study of 11,324 heart-attack survivors found that patients who supplemented with fish oils reduced their risk of another heart attack, stroke, or death. In a separate study, American medical researchers reported that men who consumed fish one or more times a week had a 50% lower risk of dying from a sudden cardiac event than men who ate fish less than once a month. However, there is some question as to whether encapsulated fish oil renders the same benefits as a serving of fish.

Calcium (1,000 mg) adds strength to bones and teeth and is needed for normal functioning of the skeleton, heart, smooth muscles, and nerves. A daily supplement is recommended to prevent loss of bone and the osteoporosis that comes with aging. Resveratrol (50 mg), extracted from grapes, helps to prevent the blood clotting that can promote a

heart attack and reduces the risk of plaque formation that invites Alzheimer's. Also, resveratrol is
thought to limit the spread of cancer cells and helps
prevent insulin resistance, a precursor to diabetes.

You'll readily agree that my food choices are unconventional, and not likely to delight a chef or find
speedy acceptance in a restaurant. But then, they've
been selected to meet an unconventional goal —
the ability to pursue health-promoting activities at
an advanced age. And what they are doing for me,
they can do for you.

4

Free Tummy-Tuck Performed on Your Kitchen Table Without Anesthetic

Be as lean as possible without becoming underweight.
— American Institute for Cancer Research

Let's Hear It for the Bacterial Multitude

Do you like gardening? I certainly hope so, because you've got a small garden of 100 trillion microbes in your stomach, all jostling each other to serve you better. (This adds numerical majesty to the estimated 10 trillion cells in the human body itself, and the conversation-stopping detail that each of us is nine-tenths bacteria and only one-tenth human.) Each bacterium — an enlarged version of which you wouldn't want to meet on the street — is busy extracting nourishment from the passing parade of food you send down, and it cries out for your constant attention.

We might laugh this off as trivia, except there's an ominous note to it all. The flora in your gut-garden determines what diseases you are (or will be) susceptible to, such as asthma, heart disease, autism, obesity, or allergies. More worrisome still, these microbes influence your daily conduct and the way you respond to challenges.

It's a fact! Studies conducted at Stanford University's Center for Genomics and Personalized Medicine have revealed the surprising impact of stomach bacteria. Your gut flora has been found to influence your behavior far more than your brain does. Worse, intestinal bacteria create small molecules called metabolites, which can reach the brain and alter its effectiveness. This puts a new spin on what mood- and health-altering edibles we should or should not be swallowing.

To fit this important detail into our puzzle of health, weight loss, and disease control, we must recognize that there is only one unfailing cure for most illnesses: the human immune system. But it has to be in top working order. Recent studies show that the gut flora has a surprising ability to boost the power of the immune system — a finding that has reawakened medical interest in a fourth-century Chinese procedure called "yellow soup" (which is, ahem, a fecal suspension) as a remedy for severe diarrhea. (Don't think about it too much.) Recent medical tests have shown that when antibiotics prove ineffective and may even have rendered the stomach biome ineffective, fecal transplantation is the only unfailing cure for cases of C. difficile.

Everyone knows (or has heard whispered) which popular foods are busy preparing a grave for you. They are the fatty, salty, sugary, fast foodstuffs — tasty, yes, but unfriendly to your body. The glaring truth is that highly sugared soft drinks, French fries, burgers, and fatty barbecued meats weaken your immune system and set you up for diabetes, high blood pressure, excessive weight, cancer, and, alas, an earlier — possibly unpleasant — departure from the planet.

Fat

Because entomophagy (insect-eating) isn't yet fashionable in Western countries, we eat four-legged animals raised solely for an assisted one-way journey to our plate — at least, some of us do. Others don't, and they're called vegetarians (cattlemen call them other names, best omitted here). But meat, whether it be hoofed or winged, comes burdened with problems, the first being the saturated fat it contains. The second is the substances that have been injected into the creature or added to its food to keep it healthy, medications that are then ferried into the human system with scant regard for what eventual effect they might have on the diner.

Trans fats, found in small amounts in some foods, come in large quantities with packaged foods, because of a process called partial hydrogenation. This type of fat also increases the risk of cardiovascular disease. But wait! While fat is usually fingered as the culprit in the battle of the bulge, that condemnation is only partially justified. After all, the body needs the essential fatty acids (EFAs) linoleic acid and alpha-linolenic acid. The body can't produce them, so they must be obtained from food.

Fat serves a second important service by carrying the fat-soluble vitamins A, D, E, and K around

our body. Fat also maintains healthy skin and promotes good eyesight and brain development in ba-
bies and children. Too little fat invites dry skin,
thinning hair, muscle cramps, and poor sleep.

Regrettably, the major failing of fat is its heavy
caloric content. Whereas sugar has four calories per
gram, fat has nine, so it's easy to quickly ramp up
your mealtime calories. But it's a mistake to equate
dietary fat with body fat. You can get fat eating carbohydrates and protein, even if you eat little dietary fat. Excess calories from any food — not just
fat — are what cause weight gain. (A gram isn't a
well-understood quantity of weight, so it might be
of some help to know that a Canadian twenty-five
cent coin weighs 4.45 grams, and the equivalent US
quarter weighs 5.65 grams.)

Salt

Salt increases blood pressure, which is the leading
cause of cardiovascular disease, heart attack, and
stroke. The American Heart Association recom-
mends that we eat less than four grams (one tea-
spoonful) of salt per day. However, North Americans
consume *ten* grams of salt per day, an amount that
favors chronic kidney damage, stomach cancer, and
osteoporosis. Most of the salt eaten comes from
packaged and restaurant foods (77%), while 11%
comes from cooking and table use.

Sodium and potassium have opposite effects on
heart health. Whereas salt (sodium) intake increases
blood pressure, potassium relaxes blood vessels and

decreases blood pressure. Our bodies need far more potassium than sodium each day, but the typical North American diet provides just the opposite. The solution? Eat more fresh vegetables and fruits, which are naturally high in potassium and low in sodium. Eat less cheese, processed meat, and other foods that are high in sodium and low in potassium.

Sugar

Sugar contributes its own deadly arrow to the heart. From the slash of a machete in Brazil to the delicious glistening white crystals on your kitchen table, sugar brings a rare allure into our lives — plus obesity, type 2 diabetes, cardiovascular disease, dementia, macular degeneration, and, ah yes, tooth decay. A 2013 study in the *Journal of the American Heart Association* displays strong evidence that sugar affects the pumping mechanism of the heart and increases our risk for heart failure. And, as is obvious if you look around, sugar promotes belly fat. Adolescent obesity rates have tripled in the past thirty years. Researchers have difficulty verifying the other perils of sugar because they can't find a non-sugar-consuming population to serve as a control!

If, as hinted, there is unhealthy cargo aboard the good ship *Lollipop*, just how dangerous is sugar to our health? Dr. Robert Lustig, a professor of pediatrics at the University of California at San Francisco, considers sugar a "toxin," even a "poison." Yet who among us isn't addicted to this most pleasant taste?

Manufacturers of all sorts of edibles and drinks boost sales by unconscionably baiting their products with sugar. Consider this: would you just sit down and eat eleven teaspoonfuls of sugar? You would if you were eating a Mars bar. You could aim lower, of course, with a Snickers bar or a can of Coca-Cola or Red Bull, each of which contains seven teaspoons of sugar. And some breakfast foods are so loaded with sugar they might justifiably be called candy rather than food. Kellogg's Froot Loops contains more sugar (41%) than it does wheat: sugar is the first item listed in the ingredients on the package. People actually buy this product and feed it to their children! Other brands of cereal gradually spiral down in sugar content until you reach Cheerios, which has just 1.1 teaspoon of sugar per hundred grams of product. But Shredded Wheat takes the day, with just one-tenth of a teaspoon of sugar per hundred grams.

Of course, we get sugar naturally from many of the fruits and vegetables we eat. For each hundred grams (3.5 ounces) of various fruits, we scoff down the equivalent of 2 teaspoonfuls in a peach, 2.2 in a kiwifruit, 2.5 in an apple or pear, and 3 in a banana. Fructose — the type of sugar in fruit — doesn't stimulate the production of insulin, and the body processes it differently than sucrose (plain sugar). Though fruit does have nutritional value, eating too much fructose will introduce new problems, such as increased blood pressure and the production of uric acid, which promotes gout.

Sugar is a carbohydrate. As such, it's often accompanied by other villains masked in various fattening disguises and tantalizingly packaged by food processors. Think cookies, honey, soft drinks, breads and crackers, jams and other fruit products, and pasta. Though carbohydrates provide energy, they're not an essential nutrient for humans. However, dietary fiber — which is supplied by indigestible carbohydrates — is essential for a healthy life. Beans, tubers, rice, and fresh fruit contain much lower amounts of carbohydrate.

Dairy Products

Now what could possibly be wrong with milk, when from cradle to grave we hear about the life-supporting benefits of dairy products (and eggs)? We do indeed, but those benefits are being touted by various producers' associations, which are interested not in your health but in continued brisk sales of their products. Here's the truth: Researchers have found a strong association between dairy lactose and ischemic heart disease (*ischemic* means restriction of the blood supply), as well as bladder, prostate, colorectal, and testicular cancers. Dairy fat is loaded with various toxins and is the main source of our exposure to dioxin, a highly toxic chemical compound.

Gone Fishing

When I think of the surprising (and regrettable) afflictions we can suffer because of a fairyland ignorance and unconcern about the foods we eat, I'm reminded of the fish pond that used to be found at fairs. Perhaps you remember going to a fair as a child and seeing among the colorful carny stalls one that had water flowing along in a trough, where for a small sum you could fish for submerged items that flowed past. The tag you caught indicated what prize you had won.

The health that each of us "catches" often seems to be acquired in a similarly random way. In a sense we are all fishing. Your neighbor's child pulls up attention deficit disorder or autism; a relative reels in anxiety or depression; others end up with Alzheimer's; and so on. But there's a major difference in our game, because we can increase the odds favorably toward pulling up a beneficial "sur-prize." We do this by strengthening our immune system, which, when loaded with suitable nutrient ammunition, has phenomenal health-rendering power.

As mentioned at the beginning of this chapter, weight loss isn't the primary goal here. I'm intent on marshaling your innate healing ability so that you will live a long and healthy life. However, oddly enough, by eating the foods that achieve this desirable goal, you can't avoid losing weight. Sorry, it can't be helped; that's the way it is. It's like tiptoeing into a weight-loss program by the back door.

I can well understand that anyone observing my current food choices might think, *If I have to eat like that I'd rather stay comfortably cuddled in my fatsuit and face the consequences.* I realize that giving up the food preferences of a lifetime is difficult, but bear in mind that the edibles I've listed were alien to me at one time. They aren't the foods I ate as a child — just thinking of the bacon and eggs, fried sausages, and steak and kidney pie makes me salivate. Nor did I switch to healthful foods all at once. As I learned the nutritional benefits of this or that food, I added it to my meals. And as I learned the health-depleting hazards of other edibles, they were dropped.

Circumstances in your life may oblige you to make a quick, drastic switch to nutritional foods, or at least wish to. But more than wishing is needed. Put autosuggestion to work for you or, as a last resort, willpower — which, according to research, each of us has in varying amounts. Surprisingly, the strength of one's willpower has been found to be linked to events early in life that favored or thwarted the development of a strong will.

Do you like stories? I think you'll enjoy this one. If A. Conan Doyle were penning the details as a vehicle for Sherlock Holmes, he might call it *The Intriguing Case of the Two Marshmallows*. Ready? In the 1960s, a team at Stanford University tested hundreds of four- and five-year-old children. They brought each child into a private room, sat them in a chair, and placed a marshmallow on the table in front of them. The researcher then offered the child a deal, saying he was going to leave the room, and if the child didn't eat the marshmallow while he was away, he or she would receive a second marshmallow. But if the child ate the marshmallow before the researcher came back, there would be no second marshmallow. The researcher then left the room for fifteen minutes. A movie camera recorded the children's facial expressions, which were often comical in the extreme. Some ate the marshmallow as soon as the researcher closed the door. Others wiggled and bounced and scooted in their chairs as they tried to restrain themselves, but eventually they gave in to temptation. A few of the children did manage to wait the entire time.

Published in 1972, the study became known as the "Marshmallow Experiment." However, the most interesting part came years later. The researchers followed each child for more than forty years. The children who had been able to delay gratification and waited to receive the second marshmallow ended up having higher Scholastic Aptitude Test (SAT) scores, lower levels of substance abuse, a lower likelihood of obesity, better responses to stress, better social skills as reported by their parents, and generally better scores in a range of other life measures.

Fortunately, a breath of fresh air comes from McMaster University, where studies have shown that willpower is alterable, and that any form of self-regulation is really an exercise in willpower. By constantly challenging yourself to resist a piece of chocolate cake, for example, or forcing yourself to perform some arduous task, you can increase your self-regulatory capacity. Willpower, like muscles, can be strengthened by appropriate exercises, so there is no need to be chained forever to an early weakness.

Knowing now that our failings are limited — and can even be reversed — only a pessimist would fall back on the comforting word *can't* to avoid switching to nutritionally improved meals. *Can't* gathers around itself an unassailable shroud that makes almost everything impossible. It's a defeatist attitude. It's like tightrope-walking across the Niagara Gorge wearing a wetsuit.

First and foremost, of course, the fast foods have to go. That isn't easy, I know. We've become so accustomed to expect piercingly delightful tastes with our food that they seem bland if they're not spiked with salt, sugar, vinegar, and a variety of spices. But it's the two-marshmallow caper again, isn't it? There they are, spread out in front of you: the steak, hamburger, french fries, colas, and fried chicken for you to devour. But if you succumb, alas, you forfeit good health and shorten your life.

Eliminating fast foods needn't be done abruptly. Just taper off. Escape the habit of always pandering to your stomach's "gimmes." While that contest is on, try adding one or other of the healthful foods I've described. And, of course, there's also autosuggestion to help you. For example, try this proclamation: "I hate spinach and I'm not going to eat it! . . . On the other hand, perhaps I could eat just enough to cover a postage stamp. It probably wouldn't kill me. Other people eat spinach and survive. . . . I'll put the matter out of my mind. At suppertime I may be overcome with a wild notion to be adventurous and eat a small portion." You get the idea: jolly yourself along; let the idea sit; forget about it. And come suppertime . . .

Subscribe to periodicals that keep you posted on the latest health news. Consumer Reports' *On Health* provides such information. And, for a more profound understanding of nutrition and health, read *Eat to Live*, by Joel Fuhrman, a most important book and one that I continue to study.

5
Laughter Is Truly the Best Medicine

I n the 1950s, *Reader's Digest* introduced its feature "Laughter, the Best Medicine," which became a long-running presentation of amusing stories thought to promote health. But did it? Proof was scanty until Norman Cousins wrote *Anatomy of an Illness.*

Cousins's book disclosed how, in 1964, he contracted ankylosing spondylitis, a rare disease of the connective tissues. Told that his chances of survival were one in 500 and that he had only a few months to live, Cousins checked himself out of the hospital and, though still bedridden, began a program of self-medication. He obtained a movie projector and spent hours watching comedies that included Marx Brothers films and the TV show *Candid Camera*, a routine that he complemented with massive doses of vitamin C. "I made the joyous discovery that ten minutes of genuine belly laughter had an anesthetic effect and would give me at least two hours of pain-free sleep," he reported. "When the pain-killing effect of the laughter wore off, we would switch on the motion picture projector again and secure another pain-free interval."

Cousins died in 1990 — twenty-six years after his predicted death. Can it be proved that laughing added those years to his life? It's uncertain. The trouble is that double-blind tests can't be conducted for proof. We can't take two groups of dying people and have one laugh and the other cry and see who lives the longest. However, experiments conducted at various universities since Cousins's time have substantiated his belief.

For example, research at the University of Maryland found that humor protects against heart disease by dilating (expanding) the inner lining of blood vessels — the endothelium — thereby increasing blood flow. And studies at the Loma Linda School of Medicine prompted the researcher to state: "Our findings show that the physiological effects of a single one-hour session viewing a humorous video appear to last anywhere from 12 to 24 hours in different individuals. This leads us to believe that by seeking out positive experiences that make us laugh we can do a lot with our physiology to stay well." By improving our body's immunity, laughter combats a host of chronic diseases, among them bronchitis, the common cold, rheumatoid arthritis, and allergies. By strengthening immunity, it may also be a supplementary measure in the control of AIDS.

The studies conducted and conclusions reached at various universities may be interesting, but they don't serve you in any way. If humor is really a curative force, as research indicates, how can we divert its healing power in your direction?

No News Is Good News

But wait — there's a fly in the healing ointment that we must first remove. I'm speaking of depressing matters that envelop you every day: those unpleasant yet often fascinating messages of gloom and doom known as the daily news. Perhaps you haven't thought about it, but the sordid stories presented by the media (who's killing or forsaking or swindling whom) jeopardize your enjoyment of a sunny disposition, which is a known powerful contributor to health. News stories are, therefore — with rare exceptions — toxic.

Let's consider how they affect you, by degrees. Suppose a good friend is grievously injured or dies. Such an unpleasant event would certainly set you up for a few bad days. But if the friend were one you hadn't seen for several years, the event would be less depressing, right? And if the injured party were someone you didn't know at all, you would feel less sadness, although you'd still experience an empathetic hurt, because we're just designed that way. A busload of children goes off a cliff in France; window cleaners in New York fall forty floors when their scaffolding collapses; a berserk gunman slaughters a group of visiting missionaries in Peru — these are the sorts of events that news reporters pour into your ears every day. And with a vast selection to choose from, there are scant limits to the tragedies and wickedness they can slither past your eyes.

Regrettably, news reporting snares everything in its net — both the calamitous and the trivial — and newspapers lend status and grandeur to trivia by proclaiming it in one-inch letters on their front pages. TV reporters similarly tout "breaking news" in their efforts to bestow importance and gravity on events simply because they are happening at that moment. This morbid form of entertainment can't be regarded as anything nobler than neighborhood, municipal, national, or international gossip. Most of the time that's what news is: sheer gossip!

What is served by your hearing about — and distantly suffering over — tragedies that can only reduce your happiness? You can't right the wrongs that have been committed or breathe life back into the victims or comfort their relatives and friends. Such gratuitous misfortunes infect you with a subliminal belief that life really isn't all that pleasant. Too many of these frightening reports will have you looking over your shoulder every time the wind rustles the leaves.

Woeful experiences trigger depression, foment sadness, and diminish happiness. Am I suggesting that you tune out the news? Yes, unless of course it plays an important role in your current lifestyle. For everyone else, though, to whatever extent you can minimize your exposure to unpleasant matters, you will advance your health.

Is there nothing good to be said about news reports? Ah, yes. They confirm — with screaming clarity — how fortunate we are to escape the afflictions endured by so many around the world. People who presume to be religious might well offer frequent thanks to their deity of choice for the opulent lifestyle they are fortunate enough to enjoy. Meanwhile, the irreligious can reflect on their luck at being resident in an affluent, reasonably safe part of the world. There's also an unexpected end run around the problem of news. Type "good news" into your search engine and you'll learn about heartwarming events that have taken place all around the globe. Be prepared, though, to shed a tear or two.

Money for Nothing?

Let's turn sharply down an avenue of fruitless ambition that nevertheless fascinates many. Ask people what would make them happy and they'll often answer, "Money." Granted, if it's a cold evening and you're lying on a hot-air grating, reading this book by the flickering beam of a flashlight, you have a problem that this work isn't designed to handle (though I could ask them to turn up the heat). For everyone else, though, money — even great wealth — often represents a futile pursuit of happiness, a yellow brick road that leads nowhere.

Consider that wealthy folk must endure most of the problems that everyone else faces, such as having to deal with others who can be forgetful, incompetent, discourteous, or all three. And costly possessions can bring a surprising array of worries. Whereas you might be troubled if someone dinged your car's fender, you could endure a never-ending succession of problems with your multimillion-dollar ocean-going yacht and its crew, vandals, port authorities, customs inspectors, and so on. And your private 747 jet airliner would add another multitude of worries and concerns.

Being wealthy provides its own burden of responsibilities and anxiety in managing and hanging on to your money. Think of the richest people in the world. Do they smile more effusively or more often than the sunny people you encounter every day? A particularly chastising confrontation with wealth can occur when riches are acquired suddenly. Type "lottery horror stories" into your search engine if this detail interests you . . . uh, preferably before buying your next lottery ticket.

Benjamin Franklin wrote sagely of the matter: "Human felicity is produc'd not so much by great pieces of good fortune that seldom happen, as by little advantages that occur every day." To which, unbidden and with audacity, I add: "and there is often twisted humor to be found in the way inanimate objects seemingly conspire to thwart one's progress." It's true, isn't it, that adversity sometimes generates its own form of bent humor. You drop something and, picking it up, bang your head, causing you to drop another item, which rolls into an inaccessible corner. You can grimace, but you might as well laugh — as I usually do (though the laughter is often seasoned with an oath).

Smiling All the Way to the Bank

Here's a surprise bonus for a cheery demeanor: smiles have been found to possess a dollar value. A team of researchers at Washington State University found that telemarketers who smile into a mirror when they are making their calls sell 17% more. And waiters and waitresses who put on a happy act make 27% more in tips.

Getting technical for a moment, there are two types of smiles. The smile we make for formal photos is one type — a false, unemotional smile achieved by tugging the corners of the mouth upward. Then there are the smiles we give to our friends and loved ones, which, in addition to raising the corners of the mouth, raise the cheeks and form crow's feet around the eyes. If you want to impress someone with your knowledge of the subject, mention that the genuine emotional smile is called a Duchenne smile, named after the French neurologist who first studied the matter.

Having verified that laughter has a proven powerful healing force, and having examined the doleful influence of news stories and the false promise of happiness rendered by financial affluence, let's concentrate on activities that are guaranteed to serve up, piping hot, healthful rewards for you in the form of smiles, laughter, and a sunny outlook.

Possibly the most promising curative light on the horizon is that shone by "laughter yoga," which works in the following way. You begin by chuckling. This seeds modest laughter that is advanced by comical movements and expressions (usually done in the company of others), until finally the participants are shrieking with glee. Laughter yoga groups are springing up everywhere. The practice seems strange only until you realize that TV sitcoms have been using canned laughter for decades to entice a more humorous response from viewers.

Smiles alone provide healthful benefits. Studies show that the movement of facial muscles when you are smiling sends signals to the brain that cause the release of endorphins and serotonin, two chemicals that make you feel happy. A sunny, optimistic disposition (expecting the best to happen) that includes frequent smiles is probably worth more than once- or twice-a-week bouts of laughter. Smiling is my preferred health-fulfilling catalyst, and it's easily secured. Surround yourself with smiling faces. It's easy. To illustrate —

I have a newspaper clipping of two youngsters, age two or three, posted on a kitchen cabinet door. The pair are smiling into the camera, and the sheer delight registered on their joyful faces forces me to smile every time I reach into the cupboard for an item. There's no charge for this pleasurable boost, no ticket to buy, and I'm not dependent on the presence of others or obliged to drive to some distant location. I receive several warming smiles every day from those youngsters, and each one prompts my return smile.

On my bathroom door I've posted a clever *Wizard of Id* comic strip, the humor of which obliges me to smile every time I view it. And on the wall of that same small, sacred room there's a newspaper photo of a pug dog with an absurdly long tongue lolling from its mouth that constantly prompts a grin. Then there's a real howler: a photo showing a small, ugly dog with large, sad eyes and a face only a mother could love, ears tucked back in submission, delivering a gentle, loving lick to a baby's face while the infant shrieks grievous resentment (what price love and affection?). I get a laugh several times a day from that one picture alone. (Incidentally, the photo accompanied a magazine article extolling the health benefits young children gain from early exposure to environmental bacteria.)

What price can you put on the healthful power these laugh-provoking pictures provide? Here in my own home I have, in these frequent boosts of humor, a free healing serum that keeps me buoyant and confident that I can handle whatever problems arise.

What sort of person posts photos of six different dogs on the bathroom wall? The same one who fits forty-six photos of dogs — past and present loyal, loving pals in their various amusing stages of growth, audacity, and authority — on the kitchen cabinets and walls. Unlike laughter yoga, the dog photos don't generate riotous hilarity. They simply make me feel warm and grateful for the pleasures I've shared with each of them. What might we call this lesser pursuit of humor? The influence that smiling has on brain circuitry is similar to the pleasurable effect produced by coca leaves (from which cocaine is made). So, "coca capers" perhaps?

Call it what you will, it's your involvement that's important.

Here's an idea. Try this interesting experiment as a small research project. The task? Each day, smile at three people you meet — people you don't normally smile at. Try it for one week. And remember, you're a scientist for the moment. You're not out to make friends or brighten lives; you just want to see what difference (if any) your smiling achieves. Go to it.

When you picture certain people in your mind, some are smiling and others aren't. Smiling has become a habit for some, a habit as natural as breathing. They don't have to think about smiling. For them it just happens, and frequently. We already know that habits can be formed, good ones as well as bad ones. So get busy building your smiling habit. To help you remember, tape an adhesive bandage across the back of one hand, and each time you notice it, tug your facial muscles appropriately. You'll find, with time, that smiling becomes easier for you. I've developed the habit of wearing a constant smile while shopping, partly to flush out interesting responses on people's faces — wonder, suspicion, surprise, and frequently (and more pleasingly) a return smile.

If you work at a desk, perhaps you display photos of your loved ones on it. Do you occasionally look at these pictures and smile? If not, perhaps it's time to substitute some others. Get busy collecting photos that generate a smile. Think of the recurring pleasure you'll enjoy from pictures that radiate happiness on your desk or at home, taped onto every door of your castle! You might include faces of animals, cartoons, or landscapes that stir a warmth in you and make you glad to be alive. Forget interior decorators' edicts about spotless walls and significant artworks — your health is too important. Joyful, health-promoting photos will serve you constantly. It's like having your own team of mood-elevating clowns.

What if you have to coax yourself to laugh? Well, why not? There's a saying in laughter yoga: "Fake it till you make it." In other words, smile and laugh even though you're not feeling amused, and let the laughter grow until it becomes a reality. The celebrated American philosopher William James neatly pieced it all together when he wrote: "Action seems to follow feeling, but really action and feeling go together, and by regulating the action, which is under the more direct control of the will, we can indirectly regulate the feeling, which is not." He then confirmed that the quickest route to cheerfulness was simply to act cheerful.

Make a list of comic movie scenes that made you laugh, and reflect on them occasionally. They made you laugh once and they can do so repeatedly. Jokes you've heard or read are similarly a valuable source of humor. Do you tend to forget gags you've heard? We all do. And that's a pity, because you can harvest their mirthful delight again and again. Write them down — they're gold. Writers of humor can also boost your spirits (S.J. Perelman does it for me) and promote off-balance thinking. Visit your local library. The humor section contains a bountiful selection of droll reading.

Does the desktop picture on your computer lift your mood? If not, type "desktop pictures" into your search engine and you'll find hundreds of photos offering a grander view of life. For a long time my monitor displayed a desert scene, devoid of life or any suggestion of life. I changed it to an autumn scene of beech trees, one so beautiful that it leaps out at me with a kiss of color and a hug for the eyes. What a day-brightener!

Supermarket Vaudeville

Now let's turn to that amphitheater of mirthless misery, the supermarket. There we are surrounded by produce from every part of the globe, foods that past kings and tycoons couldn't enjoy, and all available to us at affordable prices. Shoppers should be gleefully linking their arms and dancing in the aisles. Do they? Alas, no. They wander around with funereal expressions, despite the spirited voices above them shouting (I almost said "singing") to thunderous musical accompaniment. The inanity of the spectacle is overwhelming, and it ignites demonic mirth in me that prompts my favorite shopping game: comic supermarket pranks.

Here I must reveal my Jekyll-and-Hyde affliction. By nature I'm withdrawn. Those who know me well would never guess at the outrageous antics that accompany my freak transformation. (I should mention that there's no change in my appearance — no hair bursting forth from my forehead and cheeks or out of my ears, as depicted in movie productions. I continue to look quite normal.) In any case, I disclose these mischievous capers less for your entertainment than in the hope that they may prompt you to think, if not outside the box, at least a little closer to its rim.

Oh, I realize that being older grants me special license for imposing my humor on others, and more so if my "victim" is female. Still, you can make suitable adjustments for your age and sex. Here goes.

An easy starter is to stand beside someone who's sorting through the vegetables or fruit. When they finally pick one — an avocado, onion, pear, or whatever — let Hyde muscle in. I'll say, mournfully, "I was just going to take that one." The other person will smile or laugh and offer me the item. I smile back and refuse, having achieved my goal of making shopping a bit cheerier for both of us. Give it a shot.

Here's another easy one. When you're imprisoned at the end a depressingly long line at the cash register and someone falls in behind you, turn, smile sweetly, and say, "I've been saving that spot for you." At worst you'll get a tired thank-you and possibly a weak smile. But it's an icebreaker, and conversation easily follows. Perhaps you'll gain one more acquaintance to greet on future shopping trips.

Good reader, I presume that you aren't much different from my friends and acquaintances, who would be reluctant or horrified to attempt anything as brazen as what I've suggested. On the other hand, you could be my shining light: someone willing to take up the challenge. Most important, your involvement will become a proclamation announcing the emergence of a new, adventurous, outgoing you. Go ahead, screw up your courage. Try these two maneuvers. What can you lose? Remember, your health lies in the balance.

In 1939 the song "T'ain't What You Do (It's the Way That You Do It)" emerged, propelled by Jimmie Lunceford's heated beat. Though the title fractures drawing-room English, it conveys a compelling truth. Comments that might otherwise irritate people or even rate as an insult become socially acceptable when accompanied with a smile and a wink or a friendly nudge on the arm.

Perhaps you're ready to spread your wings and hop off the nest. All right, try this one: When you encounter a woman with a baby in her cart, ask, "What aisle did you get that wonderful child in?" You'll rack up a smile every time. As you gain confidence, you can move on to any of the following capers, or perhaps you'll think of others better suited to your age, manner, situation, or sex.

When someone queues behind me in a short line at the register, I'll apologetically inform them that the cashier's closing. As the person turns away in despair or disgust, I say that I'll ask the cashier to stay open just for him or her. They get the gag and I'm rewarded with a smile. If a very old shopper falls in behind me at the cashier's queue, I'll state in an authoritative voice that he or she is in the wrong line — it's for seniors only. Again, a pleased (and pleasing) smile.

While bagging my groceries across from another shopper similarly engaged, I'll reach across the barrier as if to swipe one of their items. This usually delights them. If someone approaches when I'm returning my shopping cart to the storage area and offers me twenty-five cents for it, I'll mention that it's a VIP cart and costs thirty-cents. "But look, I'll let it go to you for a quarter [adding some fabricated reason for my benevolence]." On those rare occasions when I catch another shopper smiling, I whisper soberly, "No smiling in the store, please," and we both enjoy the joke. (This extends to anyone whistling, singing, humming, or showing other signs of happiness.)

These comic thrusts fall far short of thigh-slapping hilarity. They're not prize-winning japes, but in a sense they are, because the prize they invariably win is a smile — my reward for attempting to generate humor in an otherwise pleasure-less environment. With luck, such capers penetrate the glacial void that keeps shoppers a safe, untouchable distance from one another. You might regard them as a sort of tickling with words. The object isn't to come out looking clever. The goal is to spread a little joy, to light a candle of cheer in an environment of gloom and despair. And the pleasure I ignite in others radiates back and catches me in its glow. It can do the same for you, if you try.

You don't have to rely solely on gags to initiate conversations. You might instead ask about some item in a shopper's cart ("Are those sugared crickets tasty? Is that maggot soup really nutritious?").

Because employment opportunities for ninety-year-olds are limited at the moment (discrimination?), I probably have more time available than many to engage in playful antics. But that's not an excuse for you to totally reject involvement, so unleash your inner youthful prankster. The world needs smiles — and never as urgently as in the great, glum shopping arena. Give it a whirl. You can do it. No one will punish you if your attempts at humor fall short. Like everything else, it takes a little practice. But at least get started.

Well, there it is. If you find that these capers lack subtlety or are tasteless (or, indeed, border on bad manners), it's because you're completely normal. I would have felt the same way when I was younger. But you may find that — thirty, forty, or fifty years from now — you attach less importance to what others think of you and more to what you think of yourself, and what role best suits you in the business of life. I had to win an inner battle to unleash my what-the-hell attitude, and you might have to do the same. It's your health we're concerned about. In time and with age, you may feel more comfortable practicing the slightly outrageous entanglements I've described.

Of course, if you can think of other, equally effective ways to conjure up a surf of delight that will shower both you and your intended recipient, for heaven's sake, use them. I've just detailed what works for me. It won't take blinding creativity or inventiveness to think of other, equally effective ways to link up with strangers.

Hierarchy: It's All About Rank

A word may be in order for those who have difficulty speaking to strangers. However much we may abhor the caste system of India, the fact remains that we are similarly observant of and burdened by our own social stratifications. Let me illustrate.

A good friend of mine, a medical doctor and a man of learning, spent his last years in a group care home. While he was there, my friend neither spoke to nor ate with the other residents. His food was brought to his room. When I asked him why he didn't engage in the social opportunities available, he explained that he couldn't because he was a snob. That's wrong, of course; he was being too hard on himself. His failing — if it can be termed that — was an inability to communicate easily with those who lacked his worldly knowledge and experience. In short, he couldn't manage small talk.

Readers of this book may be similarly hampered by a reluctance to speak to people they don't know or with whom they don't share common interests.

But whether you're a bank president, a movie star, or a world leader, your health carries the same value as everyone else's — it's priceless. It's far too valuable for you to simply shelve the notion of engaging in the various comical activities I've suggested. So, take a deep breath and dive in!

A neglected source of humor lies in failing to recycle jokes, amusing comments, and reactions we've witnessed. It seems incredible, but I still laugh at a one-liner told me by a nine-year-old pal when I was that age. That's eighty years ago! So rack your brain, dredge up the gags and jests that have made you laugh, and let them amuse you again. In fact, make a list of them for future replays.

The greatest source of entertainment isn't movies or live theater. It's in your head, available to you 24/7. Just liberate your brain and make it your onboard comedian. In time it will become a magnet for zany thoughts that keep you chuckling. You'll find yourself responding to absurdities with greater heart and developing virtual antennae that attract idiotic phrases, notions, and conditions. Comic events you once merely smirked at will begin to prompt laughter. I even laugh when I catch myself thinking of devious ways to escape unpleasant chores. Laughter while driving? When another driver makes what I consider a dumb move, I voice an unprintable comment and then have to laugh at my absurd involuntary reaction. In fact, laughing at oneself may be one of the richest veins of readily available humor.

To whatever extent you can, seek the company of cheerful, fun-loving people and try to avoid those who find life a burden (this can be difficult if those dearest to you tend to be glum). If you're not able to remedy their troubles, there is little point in sharing them.

Stuff and Nonsense

And now — *ta-da!* — for something completely different. That which follows was originally written for the chapter dealing with companionship. However, it sent out humorous blooms that demanded transplanting here. If you are unable to own a dog, here's your next best bet: get a stuffed animal.

Am I kidding? No, and before anyone calls in the white coats or slams this book closed, let me explain. At first I thought it might serve as an alternative source of pleasure for some folk, although certainly not for me. Then, feeling guilty about advising others to do what I wouldn't do myself, I went out and bought a ten-inch-tall stuffed sitting leopard cub. I won't rhapsodize over his appearance beyond saying that he's a charmer. This soft, furry one — named Fred, after no one in particular — has immense eyes set into his head so that they seem to follow you around the room.

Initially this was solely a tongue-in-cheek venture. But here's the surprise: strangely, by degrees, his guileless expression generated a pleasant, affectionate warmth in me. As a result, Fred and I have become the best of pals. I can't help but smile, even chortle, when I find him sitting on my pillow at bed-time. Because the caper is so nonsensical — sheer idiocy, too silly for words — I laugh at myself for being amused by a stuffed toy. Sort of a double scoop, isn't it.

But let's face facts — *can we have the lights flashing here, please?* — the warmth of feeling that one develops and bestows on another being, whether it's a child, an adult, or an animal (stuffed or live), is the same emotion in all cases. It differs, perhaps, only in intensity, and it promotes the same healing benefits. The brain doesn't judge or evaluate what caused the laughter before releasing its healthful chemicals: a laugh is a laugh is a laugh — and that's it.

And so Fred sits on my bedside table throughout the night and keeps an unblinking vigil for . . . aliens, perhaps? (He won't discuss the matter.) Get busy and shop for a suitable animal pal. No one needs to know, and you'll add smiles and health to your life. Take it from a convert.

A Sense of Humor

Most people will readily claim that they have a sense of humor when, in fact, they don't properly understand what attributes are required. Let's start by establishing what a sense of humor is *not*. It's not the ability to laugh at a joke or a comical situation. Anyone can do that. No, having a sense of humor enables one to find humor where it isn't obvious or intended, and to generate humor in situations where it isn't expected. Fortunately, this is a skill that can be developed. It takes practice, yes, and it hinges on a fun-loving attitude toward life and constant unearthing of comic nuggets.

Perhaps "fun-loving" is the most important part of the procedure: a mischievous digging through sober events for possible comic compost. If I get an idea for a gag, I'll even practice my lines in advance. To illustrate: I learned that my ears were full of wax and a doctor should remove it. Phoning for an appointment, I was told to insert mineral oil in both ears for a week before appearing at the doctor's office. Now, how could I inject humor into that?

When I arrived for my appointment, wearing a deadpan expression, I told the receptionists that someone there had advised me to insert transmission oil in my ears, so I'd spent considerable time under my car honoring their request. Absurd? Ridiculous? Childish? Yes, all three. However, this wasn't a coast-to-coast TV comedy broadcast, just an infinitesimal comic speck adrift in the field of entertainment. Most importantly, the receptionists broke up and their day was brightened.

Yes, these are strange, offbeat ideas (somewhat like drinking beer through a straw), but eventually you'll learn to tilt trivial matters off the perpendicular — as is done in judo — and give them an absurd twist while they are falling into comic place. Practice, practice, practice!

6
Hold Still, We're Working on Your Brain

There is hardly any inconvenience people won't endure to avoid thinking.

— Anonymous

What a different monster we might have seen if Dr. Victor Frankenstein's inept lab assistant, Fritz, hadn't stolen the wrong brain for the doctor's cerebral implant procedure. Lacking a brain in which the marbles rolled around in a precise and orderly manner, no amount of rejuvenation by sixty zillion volts of lightning electricity was likely to deliver laudable results. The same holds true for those of us outside Dr. Frankenstein's quaint castle on the hill, so if you'd prefer to skip Alzheimer's and other forms of dementia when you're a little older, listen up.

Studies conducted at the University of Edinburgh reveal that more than three-quarters of cognitive decline — which means age-related changes in brain skills such as memory and speed of thinking — was due to lifestyle and other environmental factors, including level of education. In fewer words, you're in the driver's seat for determining how you well you function intellectually twenty, forty, or sixty years from now. Researchers found that regular physical exercise, stopping smoking, eating primarily plant-based foods (fruits, vegetables, nuts, and whole grains), replacing butter with olive oil, avoiding salt, limiting red meat to no more than a few times a month, eating fish at least twice a week, and drinking red wine in moderation (optional) would grant you a world-class thinking organ.

Now if we could borrow your brain (figuratively speaking, of course) and place it in a jar for Fritz's groping hand to find, would Dr. Frankenstein have danced more joyfully for his new creation? I'm putting my money on a yes. Enter the new you: a newsworthy credit to the house of Frankenstein. (But if you hear a loud thumping on your door late some night, and through the peephole you see a grotesque hunchbacked figure standing there holding a bucket and an axe, don't open the door.)

To business. The science of neuroplasticity has shown that our brain is malleable and adapts itself to whatever demands are made upon it. Give it work to do and the brain strengthens. Ignore its potential, fail to challenge its inherent power, and it's like canceling a credit card — a matter studied by Norman Doidge and reported in his book *The Brain That Changes Itself.*

"Use it or lose it" — familiar words voiced repeatedly and worn to the status of a proverb — remains regrettably true. Put your brain to work or risk being *non compos mentis* in your later years. Of course, it's easier to do nothing, to dismiss the prospect of wandering in a daze around a shopping mall in your far-off elder years, and just hope your luck holds out. But that's lottery-ticket thinking again, isn't it.

Perhaps your daily employment makes constant demands on your decision-making ability. If so, good. Your employer is paying to keep you intellectually fit. But if your vocation lacks cerebral challenge, introduce a few of your own. We've already covered two highly recommended ways of increasing intelligence: proper nutrition and exercise. What else is there?

More Fun and Games

Here's a wild one for you. When was the last time you solved a jigsaw puzzle? Decades ago? A MacArthur Foundation study reveals that keeping the mind active with jigsaw puzzles and other mind-flexing activities promotes longevity and reduces our risk of mental illness, memory loss, dementia, and even Alzheimer's disease — by an amazing third.

Researchers credit these advantages to simultaneous use of both sides of the brain. The left brain hemisphere, our analytical side, sees all the separate jigsaw pieces and attempts to sort them out logically. The right brain hemisphere, our creative side, sees the "big picture," working intuitively. In exercising both sides of the brain at the same time, we create connections between the left and right sides, as well as among individual brain cells. These connections increase our ability to learn, to comprehend, and to remember. Also, completing a puzzle, or even just successfully positioning one piece, encourages the production of dopamine, a brain chemical that increases learning and memory.

Exercising both sides of the brain simultaneously allows the brain to move from a beta (wakeful) state into an alpha (dreamlike) state. The alpha phase is where we tap into our subconscious mind. Jigsaw puzzles naturally induce this state of focused meditation where connections can be made on deeper levels. Jigsaw puzzles therefore permit us to achieve a state of creative meditation.

Before you rush out and buy a jigsaw puzzle to begin solving at your desk (which could raise eyebrows around the office), go to thejigsawpuzzles.com on your computer. Select a picture and change the number of pieces to however many you want the puzzle to contain (the choice is between 20 and 500). Position the pieces for as long as you wish (or until the boss comes around), then save your partial solution for completion at a later time. Simple.

Maze games can improve concentration, attention span, and short-term memory. They help players remember small details, names, and events that occur throughout the day. Try mazes.ws to find mazes in four degrees of difficulty. At www .coolmath-games.com you will find not only mazes but games of logic, strategy, skill, and numbers; its parent site, www.coolmath.com, also offers lessons in pre-algebra, algebra, and pre-calculus. In short, there's a variety of challenging activities that can help seniors (and juniors) increase focus, concentration, memory skills, and reasoning. It isn't necessary to play games for hours on end; fifteen to thirty minutes a day — broken into smaller chunks if you wish — can generate impressive intellectual advancement.

But wait, we're not finished. According to Dr. Pascale Michelon, a research scientist at Washington University in St. Louis, "spot the difference" games — where small differences are introduced between otherwise identical pictures — provide blockbuster cerebral work. They offer a challenge of identification for the occipital lobes, while comparing spatial relationships between the objects in the pictures involves both the occipital and parietal lobes. Remembering what you have seen exercises short-term memory, involving the frontal and parietal lobes, and finally, marking down the locations where you spot a difference generates more work for the frontal lobe. And here you thought it was just fun and games!

You can also play X's and O's, checkers, chess, and word puzzle games, with the computer filling in as your opponent. Just type the game of your choice into your search engine to begin. You may remember that one benefit of learning to juggle is its ability to improve peripheral vision. In case you haven't started juggling yet, there are also games available on the Internet that present peripheral vision exercises.

Thanks for the Memories

Now for something completely different. Research shows that a particularly potent force for strengthening cerebral circuitry is to learn something new. Here's an unusual skill to start you off, and one that you might find daily use for.

At one time I was a stage hypnotist. To begin my performance — and generate the notion that I had rare and mysterious powers — I'd give a demonstration of memory. For this, I'd ask members of the audience to call out items we might buy while shopping, and I would write each one on a chalkboard opposite a number. When thirty items had been listed, audience members were allowed to call out an item, and without checking my written list, I'd tell them the number beside it. Or they could call out any number and I'd tell them the item beside it. Impressed?

It's easy. You can do it, but for brevity, we'll work with just ten items. First you need to memorize a sequence of ten items that will serve as "hooks" for recalling objects. So, learn the following. (This is the only difficult part; the rest is easy.) The item you are asked to picture for each number is similar in sound to the number, to aid remembering.

- For number 1, picture a *nun* (in the traditional black habit and wearing a wimple).
- For number 2, picture a *shoe* (any type of shoe you wish).
- For number 3, picture a *tree* (one with large branches).

- For number 4, picture a *door* (any type of door, but one you'll easily remember).
- For number 5, picture a *hive* (see the bees buzzing around it).
- For number 6, picture a *six-shooter* (an Old West handgun).
- For number 7, picture *heaven* (see any item that you might associate with this word, such as an angel with large feathery wings).
- For number 8, picture a *gate* (perhaps set in a picket fence).
- For number 9, picture a *line* (a clothesline, to which you can attach items).
- For number 10, picture a *hen* (just an ordinary white chicken).

Once you have memorized the above ten visual "hooks" and can rhyme them off easily, you are ready to amaze your friends — or go shopping with only a mental list of items. Here's how:

You need eggs. Okay, that's number 1 — picture a nun juggling three eggs. Next, cauliflower. That's number 2 — picture trying to stuff a cauliflower into a shoe (nonsense images aid remembering). Then shoelaces. Number 3 — picture dozens of shoelaces strung over the branches of a tree. You begin to see how the method works? Continue up to ten, using your remaining memory hooks to fasten the items in your memory.

To recall? Number 1 on the list of hooks is a nun. What is the nun doing? She's juggling eggs. Number

2 is a shoe. What were we doing with a shoe? Trying to ram a cauliflower into it. And so it goes.

As a bonus, of course, having now seen how to remember ten items, you'll be able to extend your list of memorized hooks to twenty, or even up to the (ahem) maestro's thirty. You may need help from a book devoted to increasing memory, of which there are many (more than I can remember, anyway). Though this memory routine employs a trick, it will still click your cerebral circuitry and snap your synapses — or whatever it is they do.

Here's another brain-energizing exercise. Do you know all the numbers on the various cards you carry around with you (social insurance, credit cards, car insurance, driver's license)? No? Wouldn't it be wise to commit them to memory, and to reap an intellectual benefit at the same time? And what about the people you telephone? We don't use phone numbers any more, we just push a button, right? Again, by actually memorizing those numbers, you engage in a valuable brain-boosting exercise.

More Brain Gymnastics

Reading books (not news periodicals) provides a surprise benefit. The text informs, yes, but because reading is a form of escapism, it relieves tension and stress, which are known to kill brain cells. Moreover, reading forces you to mentally picture the text, which entails a powerful brain exercise — a challenge that is regrettably absent when information is depicted on TV (this brings to mind the unsuspected value that early radio dramas provided). Reading strengthens imagination.

Have you a calculator? Put it in a drawer and forget it. Resist the urge to solve everyday math problems with an external device. Use the device you were born with — your brain! And if your computing skills are shaky, pick up a book of basic math problems or games and use odd moments to advance your ability. You'll find that solving math problems is really just solving puzzles. Fun!

When was the last time you wrote someone a letter, or even a note? No, I don't mean an email; I mean actually writing a note with a pen, putting the note in an envelope, affixing a stamp, and mailing it. What a surprise for the recipient! And you'd be doing yourself a favor. Studies conducted at the University of Washington show that a unique relationship exists between the hand and the brain when you are composing thoughts and ideas, an area of research known as "haptics." And cursive writing (the kind with joined-up letters) helps train the brain to combine visual and tactile information with fine motor dexterity.

Moving on, what about creative writing? Have you ever thought you'd like to write a book — a murder mystery or perhaps a romance novel? Great intellectual rewards are linked to imaginative writing. Research conducted at the University of Greifswald in Germany has revealed a broad network in which regions of the brain work together as a person engages in creative writing. Why don't we get you started right now? Here are some opening lines for you to play with:

Early evening fog was moving in at the Wheaton crossing. No trains now until 05:45, when the Linden early-bird would roar through. Abez, the station master, yawned, tore April 16, 1945, from the desk calendar and flicked off the lights. In bed quickly, he hadn't been asleep more than an hour when his ears caught the sound of — What? Couldn't be! A train approaching. With clanging bell and hissing steam, a locomotive was screeching to a lazy halt. By the time Abez had donned pants and slippers, the engine had started up and was puffing slowly away. That's when he looked out to see . . . nothing. There was no train. Yet a lone figure stood on the wet, steaming platform holding a suitcase.

Now it's your turn. Add a sufficient number of words to turn this opening into a comedy, then try again and make it a love story, and finally, make it a murder mystery. Give it your best shot before you check my suggested solutions in the appendix. No peeking until you've made an attempt.

7

Why Hitchhike? Take the Bullet Train to Dreamland

Though this chapter will hold special interest for those who have trouble sleeping, the solution to the problem will provide a rapid-transit trip to dreamland for everyone.

Sleep was easy when we were youngsters. No sooner had our head hit the pillow than we were off to the Land of Nod. But with maturity, alas, sleep can become difficult. Worries and concerns try to get into bed with us. And though broken sleep presents problems at any age, it exacts a steeper price for older people. Over the years I have developed techniques that promptly whisk me off to cloudland every night. They're easy to learn, and I believe they will work equally well for you. (Being tired makes the task easier, but it isn't obligatory.)

Telling you not to go to bed when you are worrying about some matter is as senseless as advising you not to cross busy roads with your eyes shut. While anxieties and fears may be difficult to abolish outright, they can more easily be crowded from your thoughts. How? By thinking of something else. It's a basic truth: you can't think of two things at the same time (which is why reading or watching TV while eating reduces the enjoyment of meals). No matter how tenaciously a worrying problem may bedevil you,

you can dispatch it to the recycling bin if you fasten your attention on some simple, repetitive ritual.

First, try a mantra. You may already know that repeating a mantra is a Hindu practice in which words — or just a single word — are said over and over again, aloud or mentally. And because you can't think of two things at the same time, a mantra can blot out other, undesirable thoughts. On the rare occasions when I have used this technique, I repeated the name of someone for whom I have great respect and affection. This not only banished the offending thought but released comforting and calming body chemicals from my brain.

Another, more traditional form of mental misdi-rection is counting sheep, but imagining sheep leap-ing over a fence is perhaps better suited to country folk. On those rare occasions when I find sleep diffi-cult, I count slowly in reverse from 100 down to 1 (100, 99, 98, and so on). This somewhat boring rou-tine, when coupled with relaxation, will get you aboard the dreamland express quickly.

Relaxation provides the second interest in our sleepy pursuit. Sleep is little more than a sustained state of complete relaxation. That achieved, it doesn't matter whether your eyes are open or closed; your body is asleep. Learning how to relax — promptly and totally — is easier for some than others. Acquiring this ability takes practice, which is best done during the day.

Using a Little Hocus-Pocus to Enter Dreamland

First, lie down, either on a bed with a cushion under your knees or on a reclining chair. Lift one arm up a few inches, hold it, then let it drop. Don't simply lower your arm; let gravity take care of things. If it helps, imagine you're playing the role of a corpse in a murder mystery. The detective lifts your lifeless arm, grunts, chews his cigar, and then lets your arm flop back down. When you can do this easily, try it with your other arm. Finally, lift both arms and let them flop down.

Once you have mastered this basic ritual, you'll have little trouble advancing to a full-blown flop-out. Continue your exercise by lifting one leg, holding it elevated, and then letting gravity drop it back onto the bed or chair. Try the other leg, then both legs. Finally, try all four limbs together. How else might you aid relaxation? You can picture yourself as a Raggedy Ann doll lying floppily at ease, or a wet sock, or a piece of cooked spaghetti hanging over a clothesline.

A procedure I've occasionally used for "snap naps" of fifteen to thirty minutes is to picture myself as an inflated body-shaped balloon with separate air valves for each body part. I pop open the valve in my lower right leg and feel it collapse as the air escapes. Same for the lower left leg. Next I pop the valve in my right thigh and feel the rigidity of that limb relax as the air escapes. Then the left thigh. And so it goes for the upper and lower arms,

then the stomach and chest. If you try this procedure, be sure to hear the pop of each valve and the
hiss of escaping air as each limb relaxes.

The head is the most difficult part to relax. First I
pop the imaginary valve in my forehead, then one
in each cheek. The facial muscles relax and in a
minute or so my jaw begins to sag. (Picture me, if
you will, lying there flopped out, slack-jawed,
mouth agape, looking less and less like Captain
America by the second.)

After four or five minutes my body begins to feel
numb. I can move my limbs if I wish, but I don't
want to — I'm too comfortable. If my nose itches, I
scratch it and then let the arm flop back down.
Nothing lost. After ten minutes or less, my arms,
torso, and legs feel as if they are encased in cement
— reminiscent of a gangland water burial in 1930s
Chicago. I can open my eyes, move my head, and
speak, if needed, while my body remains asleep.

There you have it. The procedure takes practice,
yes. But you'll gain a valuable skill. As a competent
flop artist you'll be able to use this newly acquired
ability equally at bedtime or for snap naps during
the day, even while sitting at your desk (but preferably not while driving).

Alternatively, you can imagine you're a skeleton
just lying there, bones held together with string. In
your mind, go around with scissors and snip the
connections at each joint. As each bone falls, hear a
suitable sound. Or you may hit upon some other
way to relax that suits you better. These days I no

longer need an elaborate ritual; I simply recline and flop into limp mode.

If you're able to accommodate afternoon naps of twenty to thirty minutes' duration, they will improve your mood, alertness, and performance. Famous flop artists included Winston Churchill, John F. Kennedy, Ronald Reagan, Napoleon, Albert Einstein, Thomas Edison, and George W. Bush. It seemed to work for them!

8
The Twenty-Four Vertebrae Blues

I t's a sad dance, with slow steps — really just a shuffle, and easily acquired. Too easily, in fact. You see it every day. Look around: elderly folk bent over as they move along, some unable to lift their eyes from the pavement. Such is the price exacted by spinal degeneration.

However, if you've been loading your plate with some of the nutritional building blocks described in Chapter 3, you're already on your way to owning a stronger, more supportive back. And that's what we all need, because our spine holds most of us together — at least the bits and pieces everyone enjoys seeing. In fact, this twenty-four-bone sequence running from your tail (yes, it's actually the remnants of a tail, called the coccyx) to your brain is what privileges you to stand erect.

When I was a youngster, there were a lot of old people. They were easily recognized by their gray or white, sometimes unkempt hair and weathered faces, often raddled by strife (the Great Depression was in full swing at that time). Sad expressions were rendered even more solemn by drab, colorless clothing, in keeping with the flickering black-and-white talkies (movies) of that day. Crutches and canes were a common sight.

No more. Today there are still lots of old people, but it's harder to see them. They've faded away — some have even vanished — into a magical world of hair coloring and styling, liposuction, lash extensions, cosmetic surgery, skin tightening, and whatnot. Today it's just not socially acceptable to look old. It's as if one would be letting down the team. But there is one age-marker that defies camouflage: a bent posture. And whether the postural slump is one of habit or of calcium loss in the vertebral bones, or perhaps both, this biomarker identifies its owner as aged quicker than a license plate. Fortunately, a hunched posture isn't an affliction that you have to accept passively.

If you have the physical bonus points of a Hercules (or an Amazon, his female equivalent), it's not for someone like me, who's mostly gristle and bone, to be telling you what to do. But whether or not you take up the routines described in this chapter, there is one set of procedures you shouldn't ignore — stretching exercises. To a large extent we tailor our own stance and posture, and if we don't, age does the tailoring for us. The result, alas, isn't always pleasing.

My own simple routine consists of touching my toes (or at least reaching in that general direction), backbends, side bends, and shoulder rotations. If you pursue no more than these four exercises — which take less than five minutes — you send a wakeup call to muscles that are often ignored. I push the exercising a little further with leaning pushups and lifting fifteen-pound weights. Nothing special or fancy, just a nod to my back muscles.

It's common knowledge that we "shrink" as we age. As our spinal discs lose thickness, we lose height. But worse, the vertebral bones (and other bones throughout the body) become weak and susceptible to fractures caused by the bone-weakening condition called osteoporosis. Such fractures can be caused just by bending over, coughing, or lifting something awkwardly.

Enough of the bad news. We're concerned here with keeping you smartly erect. What additional steps can you take that will prompt oohs and ahs when you reach the golden years? If your slouch is merely a relaxed slump, we can hoist you back up again. For older folks, this hoisting becomes an on-going procedure. The rules are simple:

- Keep your head up and centered over your spine (no poking your chin forward or up).

- Keep your chest up and your shoulders squared (don't cave in the front of your body).

- Keep your back straight (not curved forward).

The rules are easy; it's implementing them that takes work.

I take direction from the passing scene. Every time I see an older person with slumped posture, it reminds me to straighten up — so I do. And if I can see my feet when I'm walking, I know I'm leaning too far forward; so again, I straighten up. These same simple tricks can work for you too. Use them.

Falling becomes life-threatening for older folk. Too often we hear of someone taking a tumble, breaking a hip, and soon afterward leaving planet Earth. One exercise that contributes greatly to preventing accidental falls is tai chi. This Chinese martial art, as practiced in the West, promotes body balance and mental calmness. A 2011 review published in the *British Journal of Sports Medicine* reported that, in addition to lessening the likelihood of falls, tai chi promotes mental and physical health in elderly people. And a 2015 review in that same publication found that tai chi can be performed by people with chronic medical conditions (heart failure and osteoarthritis) without worsening shortness of breath and pain.

I engaged in tai chi a couple of years ago and practiced movements such as Strum the Pipa, White Stork Spreads Its Wings, and Carry Tiger to Mountain. However, it seems to me that any series of slow, planned movements that challenge one's balance will deliver similarly beneficial results, call the routines what you will (Taking Out the Garbage? Smoothing the Portland Cement?).

As I have said, engaging in tai chi has been found to reduce the risk of falling for older folk (by up to 45%). This protection eluded me when I bought a skateboard. I had marveled at the ease with which youngsters sped down the street with just an occasional thrust from one leg. *That's for me*, I thought. However, I quickly learned that stepping on the rear of the device tips the board and deposits the rider on the ground. So the kids on the street got a free, almost new skateboard. Now, with my newly acquired wisdom, I'd strongly urge anyone attempting this caper to first consult and then seek the guidance and support of a neighborly ten-year-old.

9
Company Comin' Up the Road — Get Out 27,000 Chairs!

Why start friendships with just a spark when you can start them with explosions? You probably know that if you're ever lost in the wilderness, you can make a fire by striking two stones together, aim the spark produced at tiny filaments of dead grass, and then blow on the smoldering mass until a flame bursts forth. Many friendships are formed in a similar way — a chance remark leads to a conversation, which leads to discovery of common interests, which leads to a friendly joint venture that leads to . . . You get the idea. Of course, friendships are more easily formed in this way if you are constantly "sparking" new acquaintances. Fine, but there's a quicker way to ignite friendships, and I'll show you how to use it.

But first, the problem. If you reach age ninety, you may find yourself single (if you weren't already). It's uncommon for both partners in a relationship to celebrate the dawn of their ninetieth year. Indeed, long before you reach that age, vacancies will appear in your circle of friends. Filling these regrettable voids can be difficult or not, depending on how you go about it. We'll look at ways that have worked for others and can work equally well for you.

There's greater value to companionship than just having someone to talk to. Companionship is rated highly for contributing to longevity. One authority advises that you either get married or get a dog (a suggestion that you might avoid mentioning to any present or prospective mate). It's true, though — the health-boosting influence of a mate or a dog exceeds the healing power of some doctors. Dogs provide more than companionship; they also generate laughter with their continual jockeying for a favored position, attention, and affection. This comedy expands with the number of dogs you own, and if your dog has some size and weight, it can also provide protection.

Best of all, of course, dogs oblige you to get out and walk. A dog's need for exercise impels action by its owner. It's no longer a question of "Should we go for a walk now?" Rather, "It's time to go!" (If it's drizzling or snowing, too bad; don waterproof gear.) And during your walk, you will encounter others with dogs, which usually generates a whirling carousel of animals, each vying for prominence in its own amusing way, barking for the edible treats they know I carry. Best of all, perhaps, are the friendships so easily formed with other owners.

People without dogs often stop and ask about my dogs' breeds, their ages, their names, how long I've had them, and so forth. Often they'll describe a dog they once owned and how much they miss it. I give them dog biscuits and they delight in feeding my three. The person who comments favorably on your dog and stoops to pet it may become a friend. So, if your work is such that it can be done at home, you might consider adding a little shaggy warmth to your life. When I mentioned this option to a neighbor who complained of stress (and who knew the benefits of dog ownership for reducing stress), he said that dogs were such a bother (tell me about it!). I could only wonder whether my neighbor really wanted to reduce the stress in his life or just wanted something to complain about.

All right, enough about dogs. How do you make new friends quickly? If you look back over past friendships you've formed, you'll find they resulted by chance or from an introduction by friends or acquaintances — in short, through luck. And though luck will continue to play a role in your finding new friends, we can load the dice in your favor with a three-step program than has never failed to win companions. The steps are:

1. Contact many people.
2. Learn to speak to strangers.
3. Invoke the friend-making magic of the masters.

Step I: Contact Many People

The first issue of *Psychology Today* (May 1967) featured an article titled "The Small-World Problem," by Harvard researcher Stanley Milgram. Milgram wanted to see how difficult it might be to connect two distantly situated people. Letters were distributed to several people in various walks of life, all of whom lived in one area of the United States. Each letter bore the same name: that of a person who lived elsewhere in the US. This person was the target recipient of all the letters.

Milgram asked the participants to hand their letter to someone they knew on a first-name basis who might be able to hand on the letter to someone closer to the target recipient (the mail could not be used). The goal was to see how many such hand-to-hand transmissions would be needed before the letter reached someone who actually knew the target recipient by name and could deliver it. You may be surprised to learn — as Milgram was himself — that the median number of passes, or retransmissions, was only five; this means that though some letters required more than five redirections, some required fewer. Indeed, one letter required only three such passes.

Max Gunther expanded on Milgram's findings in his 1986 book *How to Get Lucky*. Gunther pointed out that, while each of us has our own circle of friends, those friends in turn have their own circles of friends, which means that each of us is just one step removed from knowing a lot of people. "Let's suppose you have first-name contacts — strong and weak links — with three hundred people," Gunther wrote. He goes on to assume that each of these people similarly knows three hundred others by their first name. This would mean that by adding secondary links — friends of friends — to your initial number of friends, you are just one step removed from knowing a whopping 90,000 people. And this total, taken one step further to tertiary links — friends of friends of friends — can connect you with 27 million people! Gunther's interest lay in showing how closely linked each of us is to professional advantages, fame, and wealth, but his technique is equally effective for making new friends.

Perhaps you know three hundred people by their first name (I don't), but even with a smaller number of friends and associates — say thirty — you are just one step removed from knowing nine hundred people, and just two steps removed from knowing (or at least catching the attention of) 27,000 people. Of course, the speed and distance traveled of some detail in your private news circuit will depend on its interest. Suppose your next-door neighbor is Mary Jones. *Mary Jones had the hiccups for eight hours* isn't likely to travel far, but *Mary Jones is marrying the Duke of Bedlam in Westminster Cathedral next week* is likely to rattle a great distance in next to no time.

Now, whether or not we can hook you up with a prince or princess (we're short on kings and queens this month) will depend on the conversational bait we use. And here we must depend on what fascinating details you can provide and how well-known those details are to members of your personal group. Does every friend know where you were born and educated, have lived and worked, and what your special interests are (miniature trains, skiing, pottery, mountain-climbing, spelunking, or what-have-you)?

But let's stop for a moment. You may be wondering if (or perhaps how) this systematized hookup procedure really works. It's admittedly a gamble, like playing Monopoly, so let me run one past you. Picture, if you will, that your name is Alice and you are one of my thirty acquaintances. A friend of yours, Bentley (one of my extended nine hundred), says, "The new fellow in our shoe department, Androcles — Andy, we call him [one of my now newly extended 27,000] — had us over for a get-together. While I was there, I was on my way to the john and glanced into his bedroom. Guess what — he's got a stuffed lion on his bed!" You reply, "You're kidding! My friend Sidney has a stuffed leopard named Fred."

Well, there you have it. Information is transmitted, a phone call is made, and links are forged. Perhaps Andy and I meet to discuss *haute cuisine* for stuffed pets (primarily mothballs) or to plan the establishment of a Stuffed Pet Carnivore Association (SPCA). No, I'm not suggesting that you rush out and buy a stuffed leopard. But you need to cast a net of conversational hooks: distinguishing lifestyle features or associations, odd or offbeat pursuits, or possessions that are likely to catch the interest of distant folk.

The first set of links — over which you have complete control — are those with your inner circle: your original thirty, as it were. You might find an empathetic person simply in the process of increasing the size of this primary group, always bearing in mind, of course, that every new person added to your circle of friends adds nine hundred more associations to your extended clan, just two social circles distant. If members of your personal group produce an important more-distant contact, fine, but it's not something you should wait for. So let's consider how we can increase your initial circle of contacts quickly. Admittedly, the word *contacts* has an aura of business about it, which is misleading, because you're not pursuing friendships in order to make sales. Furthermore, you'll be able to render services to those you befriend as easily as you may benefit from their friendship.

Obvious first choices for meeting people are groups dedicated to your line of work or hobbies. If your special interest is normally a solitary pursuit — knitting or winemaking, for example — join a group that shares your interest in that craft. Then there's the congregation of your church (not religious? Unitarianism is an attractive choice for agnostics and atheists). Naturalist groups provide fresh-air activities such as studying plant growth, tracking fauna, and bird-watching. The golf course provides an easy way to encounter people who pursue that sport.

Colleges, universities, and local school boards offer a wealth of courses in skills you can learn or upgrade, and it's an easy way to meet a roomful of people interested in self-improvement. If you join a fitness program at the YMCA or a local gym, you can befriend others who, like you, value personal health. And there's another way you can exert energy that will guarantee several new acquaintances. How? (Look out, this is a wild one.)

What if — just suppose — you bought an inexpensive push-type lawnmower? Don't have a lawn? Not to worry; the mower is for other people's lawns. Wheel the mower down the street and, when you see a lawn that needs cutting, ask the owners if they'd mind your cutting the grass at no cost to them — that is, free. If they don't collapse in a faint or slam the door and call the police or medics, just explain that you'd appreciate the exercise (or give some other reason you feel comfortable with). The possible results are mind-boggling. You could end up with a plateful of shortbread cookies or, at the very least, an exceptionally warm thank-you. (Your efforts might even win a mention on the six-o'clock news or rate coverage in the community newspaper: "Lawn Barber Cuts Swath on James Crescent.") The odds are in your favor that among ten or a dozen such "clients" you'll meet one or two people who will add considerable luster to your life, and you'll bless the day you took on such a zany caper. Oh, and in the winter there's snow-clearing, right? All you need is a shovel and a strong back.

All right, we've established the theoretical value of gaining an extended family of contacts. The next step is to overcome the fear of speaking to strangers.

(Perhaps the supermarket capers described in Chapter 5 have already lessened your reluctance.)

Step 2: Learn to Speak to Strangers

We don't normally talk to people we don't know. Whether it's fear of rebuff, snub, or whatever, we're held pleasantly captive in our private little cones of silence (unless, of course, we're wearing earphones). For the moment, though, we're not interested in making friends, only in overcoming any natural reluctance we may have to speak to people we've never spoken to before. So remember, for now it's just an exercise.

Next time you're close to a stranger, screw up your courage and speak to him or her. What can you lose? People rarely pull a knife on others who speak to them in a non-threatening way. If you're waiting for a bus, the weather is a natural topic: "Chilly today." "Hotter than usual." "Will this rain never stop?" "They're forecasting more snow for this afternoon." (And so on.) Or ask a question. "Excuse me, could you tell me the time, please?" (You have a wristwatch, but that's beside the point.) "Excuse me, do you know if this bus stops at Warren Street?" (You know it does, but again, that's incidental.) "Excuse my asking, but where did you buy that attractive hat/coat/ purse/whatever?"

If you're eating in a café or restaurant, look for ways to send out a verbal lasso. If you sit near someone or someone sits near you, see if there is an opportunity for comment. "That speckled lizard looks delicious. I think I made the wrong choice."

An elevator ride presents little opportunity to engage in friend-making, but suppose you get off at the wrong floor *on purpose.* Earlier in the book I advised those who work or live in a high-rise to take the elevator down a few floors and climb back up again for the exercise. You could follow a similar procedure for the opportunity of exchanging a few words with someone new. Is there a receptionist or some other friendly-looking person you could greet stationed near the elevator? Choose different floors to get off on different days and find out.

A doctor's waiting room presents a special challenge. The magazines often cover matters of little interest and are usually out-of-date. So take along a few printed pieces that you would normally discard after reading — items dealing with travel, health, or other useful topics — and ask the other people waiting if they'd like to read them.

If you take a cab, see how much information you can glean from the driver before reaching your destination. "Is Vancouver your hometown? How long have you lived here? Have you been driving a cab for a long time? Have you been in any accidents?"

Volunteering provides an easy opportunity to begin communicating while also offering the possibility of establishing a valuable friendship or two. After all, you will be meeting "giving" people who are freely donating their time and effort. Community-based organizations such as the YMCA welcome helpers for

their various programs. Give some a call and see
what's available. Visit a nursing home and share a
few kind words with people who are nearer life's
end. Or you might help out at a soup kitchen or food
bank — an opportunity to get close and personal
with folks who have many more worries than you.

Candidates running for public office need volunteers to canvass, answer phones, and erect signs.
And volunteering can offer an interesting way to
learn a new skill or trade. Few enterprises will turn
away someone who is willing to work without pay
solely for the chance of learning about their business. The opportunities for volunteering are limit-
less. Just type "volunteering [your city's name]" into
your search engine. Though you may have limited
time to give to the venture, you'll find an arrange-
ment that suits you.

You're beginning to see how you can easily overcome any reluctance you may have to speak to
strangers. However, up to this point you've made
many contacts and have overcome your inhibitions
about speaking up, but you haven't necessarily
made any friends. Which brings us to the third important step.

Step 3: Light the Explosive and Stand Back
Do you know what will grab people's attention with
a grip tighter than a refrigerator magnet, making
them like you instantly and remember you forever?
Give up? Pay them a compliment.

Think. When was the last time anyone bothered to comment favorably on your manner of dress, speech, work, patience, or whatever? It's a lost art — gone, like last year's roses. But that's what makes it so easy to achieve world-class skill. You're ahead of the game before you start. You can't lose! Compliments can make you myriad friends, at no cost beyond the spoken words.

Don't take my word for it; give it a shot. Start with an artist. No, not a painter or sculptor, but the person who works in the produce department of your supermarket. Keep it simple — nothing too fancy. "You do a terrific job keeping all the items well organized and looking attractive." Well, if he doesn't drop dead from shock at someone recognizing, first, that he's human, and second, that he works hard to keep the fruit and vegetables looking fresh and desirable, you're guaranteed a welcoming smile every time you shop. So you've both gained, right?

But don't stop there. Shoppers abound, and each one provides an opportunity to work your complimenting magic. You may never be able to physically levitate anyone, but you'll be able to raise their spirits with dazzling ease.

Ah yes, but first, what do all magicians do? They practice, practice, practice. They do, that is, if they want to perform in Las Vegas. Top magicians spend hours practicing their mystifying routines until their movements become automatic. So it's obvious what you need to do, isn't it. Nudge yourself to get started. Bountiful rewards are yours for the effort.

But note: I'm not talking about flattery, which is just vocalized hot air, unworthy of your attention. You must genuinely appreciate that which prompts your compliment. If I see someone with an impressive hairstyle or wearing a piece of clothing that I truly admire, I'll tell that person so. And if the situation warrants humor, I might add, "If you ever discard that coat/hat/whatnot, let me know and I'll come and get it." They will probably walk a bit taller because of my compliment and perhaps repeat it proudly to someone at home.

Now start thinking about people you routinely encounter who genuinely rate a compliment. Next time you meet each of them, let them know they have an endearing quality that you think they display with distinction. "I've often admired the way you [do something]. I hope you'll excuse me for telling you." It's not a big deal. And don't wait for thanks; it's your gift, not theirs. Compliments are verbal flowers of delight. Distribute a few — it costs nothing. Begin tomorrow. Smile at people you normally ignore. Try it for a day or two and see what happens.

By gradually becoming more aware of pleasing attributes in others and voicing your pleasure, you'll eventually give compliments so easily they'll come automatically — and you'll harvest smiles from all sides. Nothing new here. William James said, "The deepest principle in human nature is the craving to be appreciated." And it's true, isn't it. Each of us nestled in our little corner wants to shine a light of consequence into the world. *We're here, we matter!* One of humankind's greatest desires is to be appreciated and feel important. It's this thirst for feeling superior in rank and importance that dresses officials elegantly in robes and tasseled garb with gold braid, bells and whistles, and great feather plumes of authority, all proclaiming — nay, shouting — *I'm important!*

Dale Carnegie, author of *How to Win Friends and Influence People*, illuminated our golden walkway to friendship back in 1936, when he said, "You can make more friends in two months by becoming interested in other people than you can in two years by trying to get other people interested in you." Wait! That's so important it deserves typographical emphasis:

> **You can make more friends in two months by becoming interested in other people than you can in two years by trying to get other people interested in you.**

Wouldn't it be a good idea to test his theory? It costs nothing, and the potential rewards are overwhelming.

Do you want to know a secret quick-setting mortar that cements convivial bricks into place? Dale Carnegie revealed the key ingredient in the mix:

people's names: "A person's name," he said, "is to him or her the sweetest and most important sound in any language." Using a person's name repeatedly in conversation holds their attention, right? (So next time you're in the produce department, get the attendant's name and voice it as often as possible.) Think of it: when someone remembers your name after meeting you, you feel respected and more important. It makes a positive and lasting impression on you.

And yet, despite the obvious importance of learning other people's names, how many of us promptly forget them? Almost everyone. Is there is trick or a gimmick to help in remembering names? Several.

- When someone tells you his name, immediately use it in the conversation: "Bryan's right, you know, not all lawnmowers are built the same." Or tag his name at the end of a question: "Where do you buy your socks, Bryan?"

- Have the person spell his or her name. "Is there an E at the end of your name, Anne?" "How do you spell your name, Lyudmila? Again, please, slowly."

- Most effective, though, is to write down the person's name at the first opportunity, adding any tidbit of information that was offered regarding her work, family, or interests: *Edna, born in Brussels, three children, plays badminton.*

Salespeople (and politicians) use this practice to great advantage by noting details that emerge in the conversation: *flower shop, owner, Henry, born in China, builds model planes.* By referring to their notes before a subsequent meeting, they're primed to say, "How's it going, Henry? Did you get the motor into that Spitfire you're building?" And, of course, Henry is surprised and delighted that someone is interested in the progress of his hobby.

A businesslike procedure? Yes, it is, but if we want to escape mere chance as the sole means of making friends, we are wise to go about the task in a methodical and effective way. A miniature recorder, easily carried in a pocket or purse, or the voice memo feature on your phone will permit rapid notation of such incidental matters.

Next, there is one subject that everyone is an expert on, a subject about which they will talk endlessly, given the opportunity. Can you guess what it is? Time's up. It's themselves. As long as people feel confident you're not out to sell them something, most will gladly tell you their life story. This makes conversation easy for you — all you have to do is keep asking questions. Disraeli, one of the most powerful prime ministers England has ever had, said, "Talk to a man about himself and he will listen for hours."

Your efforts have more than immediate attention-grabbing power, because the more information you gain about people, the more your own importance grows in their eyes. Think about it: the people who are important in your life (employers aside) are those who know a lot about you. So, securing more information about others will boost your informational stature, and conversations will inevitably swing around to include you, the newly arrived important person.

The Sweetness of Touch

And now for dessert. You might get a few questioning glances if you open a box of chocolates and offer them around the office, where everyone is trying desperately to lose weight. But what if I told you there's a no-calorie sweetness you can give freely, that costs nothing, is barely perceptible, and brightens people's days? Get ready . . . It's a simple touch!

Recent studies from England have pinpointed an area in the brain — a region called the orbital frontal cortex, located just above your eyes — that becomes highly activated in response to a friendly touch. It's the same area that responds to sweet tastes (such as chocolate) and pleasing smells. The researchers found that a warm touch releases a surge of oxytocin, which makes you feel more trusting and connected. A cascade of electrical impulses slows your heart and lowers your blood pressure, making you feel less stressed and more soothed. Remarkably, all these complex events in the brain and body result from just one gentle, supportive touch.

A French study found that when teachers pat students in a friendly way, those students are three times as likely to speak up in class. And in a 1976 study, university library clerks returned students' library cards either with or without briefly touching the student's hand. Subsequent interviews revealed that those who'd been touched — even if they didn't notice it — evaluated the clerk and the library more favorably. The same result was found in a study conducted with bank employees. When dealing with clients — either giving them money or taking in deposits — tellers were instructed to make certain that they touched the customer's hand ever so briefly in a seemingly accidental manner. When clients were later quizzed, those who had been touched rated the staff as more courteous and friendly.

And how about the world of sport? Psychologist Michael Kraus, of the University of Illinois at Urbana-Champaign, tracked friendly physical contact between teammates during professional basketball games, such as chest bumps, high fives, and backslaps. The study showed that the more on-court touching players engaged in early in the season, the more successful were the teams and individuals by season's end. The effect of touch was independent of salary or performance, which eliminates the chance that players were touched more if they were more skilled or better compensated.

Research conducted by Dr. Tiffany Field, director of the Touch Research Institute at the University of

Miami, shows that many forms of touch can help reduce pain, anxiety, depression, and aggressive behavior; can promote immune function and healing; and can lower heart rate and blood pressure and improve air flow in asthmatics. All this and no drug side-effects! Moreover, there are reciprocal benefits — you can't touch without being touched. In fact, although we're the ones initiating contact, we may reap the same benefits as those we're touching. A person giving a hug gets just as much benefit as the person being hugged.

So add a little health and happiness to your life — and to the lives of others — by surreptitiously touching them, maybe at the office when passing along orders or reports, or while chatting with neighbors or shopping. I manage this sometimes by helping the shopper ahead of me transfer hard-to-reach items from their cart up onto the checkout counter. A simple brushing of hands as they take the item from me, and that's it. Imperceptible physical contacts can make you seem a surprisingly friendly person, and no one will guess why.

Friendly Overtures

A quick and effective way to radiate friendliness is easily achieved just with the voice. Use public transit? Greet the driver with "Good morning" and voice a hearty thank-you when he hands you a transfer (he may faint). Repeat those words with a smile to mail carriers, and to cops too (always best to keep them friendly and on your side). Make a habit of opening doors for other people. (I find that opening doors for younger people can be amusing — women usually accept the gesture with thanks, while men will generally refuse to precede an older person.) Let a shopper with just a couple of items precede you at the cashier. If you see a couple with a camera, perhaps they'd like someone to take their photo.

Food can convey friendship, and more. A former fellow-worker showed me a hardboiled egg he had found in his lunch. Penciled on it were the words "I love you" — an affectionate reminder from his mate. When a new family moved into the house beside me, they knocked on my door, introduced themselves, and presented me with a small box of confectionaries. How nice. A lesson for all of us.

Sweets have always served as a vehicle to express affection, seemingly with sound scientific backing. The chocolate junkies among us can rejoice at data from the University of Aberdeen, in Scotland, where an analysis of 29,951 participants over 11.3 years showed that eating up to a hundred grams of chocolate every day lowered the risk of dying from heart disease by 25%. The chance of suffering a stroke also fell, by 23%. Incidentally, the levels of the beneficial flavonoids responsible for these results are higher in darker varieties of chocolate.

Social Media

Many people see Facebook as an easy way to attract prospective pals into their living room or office. It can be done, and occasionally we even read of marriages resulting from an initial meeting through Facebook. You could be that lucky too, but such successes happen so rarely they're reported as news items. What's more, Facebook and its ilk present hazards.

You could be stepping onto a tilting trestle of communication, one that, according to research at the University of Gothenburg, can prove addictive. Participants in their study grew ill-at-ease when they couldn't regularly check their Facebook accounts. And with new material being posted constantly, the participants felt they were losing out when they weren't logged in, all the while failing to realize that their involvement was now a compelling unconscious habit.

Facebook and other social media enable you to share much personal information about yourself. This can invite identity theft. Caution is needed about the privacy settings on one's account. Hackers can use your personal information to gain access to your other online accounts, or even open new ones using your identity. Obviously the benefits of social media are balanced by its disadvantages. Better by far that you direct your attention to existing friends rather than pursuing electronic beyond-the-horizon pals.

Boosting Up Friendship Two Rungs at a Time

Remember when we used to send Christmas cards? That form of greeting has largely given way to a simple email message. However, there remains one other date when our good wishes are still best conveyed by a card — or, even better, by voice — and that's someone's birthday. That's the day the world began (well, theirs did, anyway). So how can you give them a greeting on their birthday when you don't know the date? You learn it by a slightly devious method.

Buy an inexpensive annual of astrological predictions. Next, read out for a friend a few fanciful words disclosing what the annual says about you for that day. Then wonder what it says for your friend — who of course will disclose the great day he or she entered the world. If you want to excel at this art, memorize the signs of the zodiac and some of the supposed attributes of people born under each sign.

For example, Aquarius covers the period from January 20 to February 19. Aquarians supposedly achieve an intellectual pinnacle higher than all others; they are the scientific thinkers. When you've memorized the details for Aquarius, learn the other eleven signs (shown below). Here's a tip: don't try to learn them all at once or you'll become confused. Commit just one to memory each day or every couple of days. You can find characteristics for each sign in the booklet you purchased or through the Internet.

Signs of the Zodiac

Aquarius (the water-bearer), January 20 to February 19

Pisces (the fish), February 20 to March 20

Aries (the ram), March 21 to April 20

Taurus (the bull), April 21 to May 20

Gemini (the twins), May 21 to June 20

Cancer (the crab), June 21 to July 22

Leo (the lion), July 23 to August 22

Virgo (the virgin), August 23 to September 22

Libra (the scales), September 23 to October 22

Scorpio (the scorpion), October 23 to November 22

Sagittarius (the archer), November 23 to December 21

Capricorn (the goat), December 22 to January 19

With this knowledge you are now a virtual mobile birthday detector. Follow the procedure described above. You don't have to remember twelve different descriptive details. Just wing it: "I believe your sign says you're a natural leader [or a warm, dedicated individual/an exceedingly honest and dependable person/a pursuer of scholarly excellence/a spiritual guru always eager to spread happiness/anything else that pops into your mind]." Let your creative skills run riot. Most important, you now have the all-important date to honor when that day rolls around.

Imagine your friend's delight when, out of the blue, he or she receives a surprise birthday greeting from you, delivered verbally or emailed or — like frosting on the cake — via a mailed birthday card. There are few more impressive ways to honor a friendship and demonstrate the pleasure you have gained by knowing him or her.

While thanks will probably be forthcoming, thoughtful responses aren't universally rendered. Such an omission might surprise you, as Shakespeare's King Lear grievingly affirmed: "How sharper than a serpent's tooth it is to have a thankless child." However, there is another reward to be savored without having to seek those elusive thanks: one described in Lloyd C. Douglas's novel *Doctor Hudson's Secret Journal*. It's the practice of doing good deeds secretly without seeking exposure or credit, reaping instead a spiritual boost — a treasured flower for your buttonhole. *And it is.* After all, the opinion we hold of ourselves is of infinitely greater value and importance than what others think of us, right?

Now, if you have trouble spotting good deeds to perform, take a plastic bag with you when you're out and about and pick up litter. *What? That's going too far!* You didn't create the mess, so why should you pick it up? Anyway, the city pays people to handle that task (though, admittedly, service may be slow). And yet, and yet . . . the pop cans and crushed cigarette packets and foil wrappers remain, offending every sensitive person who passes.

But worse, by letting trash reign over the landscape, we miss a rare opportunity to express our personal form of *noblesse oblige* — the obligation that a socially superior individual bears toward others. We lose, in fact, a chance to disclose (quietly) that we're on nature's side. It's a hug and a kiss for the community, and you can still pat yourself on the back.

Various ways have now been described to set you up as a warm, caring human, one who will more easily win new friends. The likelihood of meeting someone with whom you might form a lasting friendship rises proportionally with the use you make of these suggestions. Lay aside this book (after you've finished reading it, of course), switch off the TV and the computer, go out into the world, and begin practicing the procedures, gimmicks, and capers that have been proposed.

Nodding in agreement that the methods described will probably achieve your desired goal isn't enough. You have to act. You get only one life and you're living it right now. Sorry, that's the way it is. So, unless you give some immediacy to your good intentions, they could end up as to-do tasks in that ectoplasmic other-world. Alas, a little too late for this one.

10
The World's Your Oyster, So Eat

In this age of specialization, scientists, engineers, and other professionals often achieve their advanced skills at the price of crowding out many other fascinating interests — which tends to make their abilities, in my eyes at least, an awesome but narrowly tunneled accomplishment.

Look around you. There is such a dazzling spectrum of crafts and hobbies to taste or to swallow whole. And because, by age forty or fifty, most of us have sufficient ability in some field to guarantee a continuing income just by harnessing up each day and applying shoulder, we can usually find the time. I'm not suggesting that anyone ditch their daily job so they can start woodcarving or coin collecting full time. No, but perhaps some of your time is being currently and casually given to inconsequential matters — such as TV viewing or reading the newspaper — when it could be devoted to a more rewarding activity.

Granted, at ninety I probably have more time than many to pursue new interests. What use am I making of the opportunity?

I'm Singin' in the Rain — and Elsewhere

When I was young, whistling, not singing, was the popular way of airing melodies. Even women sometimes whistled in those days. That partially explains why I never sang. However, when I was eighty-eight I decided I wanted to learn to sing. I played musical instruments in dance bands as a youngster (reeds mostly), which means I am sensitive to pitch (knowing when a note sounds in tune). In case you'd like to learn to sing, I'll tell you how I went about it. (Mind you, I still sound terrible, but what an improvement I've made in the past two years!)

First you need to be able to voice notes correctly. Begin by singing simple songs — Christmas carols, "Happy Birthday to You," or whatever. The song isn't important. It's hitting the notes accurately that matters. So sing the songs very, very slowly, giving full attention to whether or not you're hitting each note bang on (this is called intonation).

When you gain confidence that you're sounding the notes correctly (it may take months), gradually speed up the procedure until you can hit a sequence of notes quickly and accurately. As a bonus, you'll probably find that you're gradually becoming able to include higher and lower notes — gaining an extended range.

When, on that grand day, you can voice songs easily and in tune, there's one more difficult part to learn: vibrato (the one I'm still busy with). Vibrato is a pleasant wavy tremor given to musical sounds. If you're a dead loss at being able to embellish your musical tones with vibrato (as I was), begin by imitating the sound of a car's motor starting up and not catching: *uh-uh-uh-uh-uh-uh*. Practice this as often as you can. The months will tick by and gradually you'll begin voicing a smoother imitation of a stalled motor. It might take a year to finally secure a singing voice of sufficient quality to make people stop and applaud. It's a long haul, admittedly, but I didn't promise you a quick recording contract. (My instructions for learning to sing might make a singing teacher feel queasy, but this method worked for me.)

Off We Go into the Wild Blue Yonder

As a child I was aircraft-crazy, so of course during World War II I joined the Royal Canadian Air Force. Unfortunately I got no higher off the ground than you can jump. Finally, at age ninety, I decided to fulfill a lifelong desire to pilot an airplane. My craft of choice was a canvas-winged ultralight trike, which, as its name suggests, has a single triangular wing attached to a three-wheeled undercarriage.

A trike has no cockpit. You just sit there in the open air with no parachute and with the ground a long, long way below — which might make some people nervous. In three lessons I advanced sufficiently to taxi around the approach strips and briefly control the craft in flight.

I acquired several study manuals dealing with government air regulations, navigation, aerodynamics, meteorology, electronic communication, and just about everything short of what is needed to pilot a 747. Alas, it gradually dawned on me that, while I would eventually be free to purchase any aircraft I wished and taxi it to my heart's content, the moment the wheels left the ground, I would no longer be in complete control. That's where the government steps in. Ahem, they own the sky — and if you want to use their sky, you have to honor their requirements and secure certain qualifications.

My simple desire to hop into a plane, buzz around, and playfully barnstorm anything I wished became lost in a shredded wheat of bureaucratic constraints. When I discussed the matter with others who had gone all the way and acquired the papers, they admitted that the cost of flying prevented their enjoying the air freedom they had worked so diligently to obtain. And so my dream of flying, having completed a circuit, ended up smoothly back on the runway. Now, alas, it is once again just a longed-for activity that I can pursue only while dreaming.

It's Magic!

Would you like to shine with blinding effulgence at any group gathering? Here's what you do: add a magical component to your presence — i.e., perform magic. Wait, I'm serious. These days neither practice nor skill is required to astonish friends, acquaintances, and colleagues, and they'll think you're really something special. (I captivate children at a private school every time I visit.)

A little background. Gone are the days when you had to practice for hours in front of a mirror to perform mystifying manipulative procedures, prestidigitation, sleight of hand, and a gamut of dazzling effects. Today everything is often done for you. Clever gimmicks and gadgets are readily available that require no practice. With such devices I'm able to perform mind-blowing tricks that any seven-year-old (make that six-year-old) could repeat in two minutes if they had the material.

You can do the same. There are several purveyors of magic materials that can easily be purchased through the Internet. (I use Penguin Magic and find them helpful and fair.) Or you can visit a magic store, where the attendant will baffle you, sell you the baffling material, and then send you off to baffle the world.

A World of Possibilities

I've already mentioned my near-death caper with a skateboard. Don't try it unless you're a lot younger than ninety. But is there some other physical activity you've always wanted to conquer? How about swimming? Perhaps now is the time (I didn't learn to swim until I was fifty). Perhaps you sing. Glee clubs usually welcome new members.

Join an amateur theatre group and audition for a part. If you don't get cast, fill some other role in the production. Help with props, costumes, or scenery, for instance.

You might write a book — as I'm doing here. People often claim they have "one good book in them." Could that be you? Get started. You've probably experienced (or endured) events that would interest others — if only your grandchildren. Maybe you didn't go over Niagara Falls in a barrel or climb Mount Everest or cross the Atlantic Ocean in a canoe, but you *thought* about it, so tell others. Vanity publishers await eagerly to apply all the trimmings (editing, design, artwork) to your writing and turn it into an impressive opus, which they'll then distribute for you. (For an illuminating critique of this form of publishing — one that reveals its several dangers — type "friends don't let friends use vanity publishing" into your search engine.)

Alternatively, you might write a book about other people. Visit a retirement home and chat up some of the residents. You may be surprised at the fascinating involvement some older folk can report of early events in your city or town. Write them up, produce a book, and put a price on it sufficient to cover the printing costs. (You don't need a publisher. Most printers can turn out an attractive market-quality book.)

Of course, the Internet offers an abundance of suggestions for branching out your interests this way or that. Bridge clubs provide an excellent way to meet others while boosting cerebral activity. The basics are easily learned. (An Internet program presented by Richard Pavlichek caught my eye and has prompted me to begin learning the game.)

Night courses offered by community colleges, universities, and school boards permit you to study for an educational credit or simply to satisfy a fascination you may have with some subject. And, of course, academic studies provide intellectual stimulation as a bonus. Language learning is popular. Are you hoping to visit some foreign country in the future? Best that you have at least a rudimentary grasp of that country's language. Many colleges offer discounts to retirees above a certain age.

Alternatively, you may have special knowledge of a field that interests others. If so, you could teach: offer a free course at your local library or community center.

Are you musically inclined? With so many musical instruments to choose from, there's sure to be one that fascinates you. Visit a music store and discuss your interest with an expert.

Natural Wonders

One of the best — and most interesting — part-time pursuits is volunteering. Though already mentioned earlier, volunteering rates a revisit because of its flexibility and wide range of application. You can select any degree of involvement to suit your schedule or interest.

You might consider helping at an animal shelter, or even take home a pet that needs special care. (*Hmm, he's back to dogs again.*) The benefits that accrue to your personal well-being from caring for a pet are well documented. If you live in housing that doesn't allow pets, what about pet-sitting in someone else's home? Or you might walk and feed their pet and give it some playtime. People have even given up regular daytime jobs to pursue this healthier way of life.

While you're mulling that one over, why not take in a few houseguests? I don't mean humans, I mean potted plants. Research conducted at the University of Bonn reveals that 99.9% of a plant's biomass actually behaves in the same way as an animal. Studies show that plants keep time, know themselves, count, distinguish kin from strangers and competitors, explore for the best patches of soil and sun, and chemically warn of (and ward off) enemies. All this and they're not able to speak (not yet, that is).

Better still, the American Horticultural Therapy Association claims that gardening may reduce blood pressure. Worth a try, isn't it? Biologists contend that a plant's evolutionary arsenal is far more complex than an animal's because it's immobile. Plants evolve ingenious mechanisms to survive drought, pests, and predators. Research conducted at several universities proves that plants display animal-like behavior. First, they are constantly communicating with one another (in their own language); second, they are continually foraging and hunting for food, both above and below ground; and third, they dispatch messages — via aromas — to attract predators that will devour the insects attacking them. Furthermore, plants are continually moving (though rarely as quickly as the insect-eating Venus flytrap). Finally, a study conducted in a Douglas fir forest revealed that plants share resources and are more likely to do so for their offspring.

There's been talk that plants react to human touch, words, and thoughts. Is it true? I don't know, but it would make an interesting research project for you. And if you develop a nine-foot carnivorous Venus mantrap, you might get asked onto the late-night talk shows — especially if you can train it to devour a two-hundred-pound fruit fly.

While discussing the smaller life forms, I must reveal the growing respect I've developed for all living things. The life led by a toad or a mouse or a butterfly doesn't appeal to me, but I recognize that the creature's lowly existence is important to it. When I was younger, I could slip a worm onto a fish hook without a second thought. I couldn't do that now. Worms too have their own sacred life to lead, as do all insects, and it's not for me to interfere with their existence. Except those that come into my home . . . then their lives are forfeit. *Zap!*

11
Showbiz in the Home

It's all comes down to attitude, doesn't it. You may remember that when David confronted the giant Philistine Goliath, he didn't turn and run for the hills, as most of us would have done. He took a stone from his pouch, fitted it into his sling, aimed, and . . . well, made history (if we're to believe the tale). The lesson here is that we can't solve problems by running away. A winning attitude can achieve wonders. (Though there's no guarantee it will work, of course. What if Goliath had sneezed and thus avoided David's stone, then dispatched the youngster to a hero's grave? With that speculative thought, we'll exit the story.)

To some extent we pick the cast for our day's drama. As Shakespeare said, "All the world's a stage and all the men and women merely players." He was right. We each have a "wardrobe" of personas. Which outfit will we wear today — happy and optimistic or sour and pessimistic? We determine what sort of person will step outside our home each morning.

How you act influences how you feel. It's William James's assertion all over again. So if you've ever thought you'd like to act, here's your chance. Give an Academy Award performance by filling the role of the person you want to be for the day — always bearing in mind that, as mentioned in Chapter 4, our gut flora plays a part in establishing both how we think and how we feel. (If you find it difficult to radiate a sunny mood, perhaps you should examine the food you're eating. Maybe the bacteria in your gut are trying to send a message: *Send down the high-fiber food we need and we'll stop being grumpy.* Time to review Chapter 4?) In any case, it gives a new twist to Abraham Lincoln's words, "People are about as happy as they make up their minds to be" (perhaps that should be "as happy as their gut flora permits them to be").

Here's the bottom line: It isn't how wealthy you are or the social prominence you've achieved that makes you happy or unhappy. *It's what you think about your situation.* Personal advantages play no part in the delight. You may already have noticed that the wealthy, famous, and powerful appear to be no happier than the clerks at your supermarket. Take two people who own approximately equal assets, advantages, and benefits. One may be happy and the other miserable. Isn't that true? We all have a choice. Pick a winner: the radiant, optimistic, fun-loving you.

We are living in the fabled land of milk and honey, enjoying so many blessings that we should be happy around the clock. Surprisingly, the greatest pleasure you can secure — the greatest currently available to you (and *free*) — is to recognize your present good fortune. Nothing matches it. If you have health, vigor, food, and shelter, you are wealthy right now. What ailing multimillionaire wouldn't trade his riches to escape an oppressive illness and gain your health? But he hasn't enough money to buy your health. Its value is beyond price.

12
Welcome to Ninety

Problems you previously solved with muscle must now be solved with brain.

Most readers are probably still on their way to reaching ninety, so let's look at a few things to be enjoyed when that great day arrives. If you've already made it, welcome. Sit down while I address the juniors.

Leading the parade of life adjustments are nocturnal trips to the bathroom — an indelicate topic, true, but you'll find that the later years introduce several indelicacies. And for those who can't make the nightly trips successfully or quickly enough, there are products available to meet this failing. (Home medical supply stores offer a surprising range of items to ease this and numerous other complaints.)

Partial loss of hearing will introduce you to an amazing array of supplemental hearing devices. Long gone are the days when hearing aids merely made sounds louder. Today's tiny appliances amplify only those frequencies that your ear no longer registers well (loss of the higher frequencies turns everyone's speech into a mumble). Insensitivity to smells will render you unable to detect body odor and, regrettably, some flowers. And, of course, you may endure some unpleasant physical impediments, for example, a touch (or a wallop!) of arthritis.

Finally, an even more delicate matter. If the pre-pubertal youngsters will briefly leave our circle, we'll discuss sex. Thank you. Now, with the door locked and the shades drawn, we, uh . . . well, actually, it turns out that the sexual appetite and its pursuit are highly individualized. (Though I think George Burns described the situation aptly for many men when he said, "Sex at age ninety is like trying to shoot pool with a rope." Women, being possibly more discreet, haven't broadcast any similarly revealing statement.) To secure an enlightened prediction of your future sexual ability at ninety, you may have to consult a Ouija board.

Mind you, these afflictions don't hit you slam-bang all at once. You acquire them (or don't) gradually, over a period of years. Furthermore, it isn't all gloom and doom for older folk. You'll find that strangers are more courteous; they'll open doors for you and smile. Even more important, you acquire elasticity with the law. Police officers are reluctant to chastise (much less ticket) people old enough to be their grandparents. And you're free from chasing the dollar. If you haven't got a nest egg to finance your basic needs, the government will at least see that you don't starve.

The contents of the public library are yours. All those books you wanted to read but never found time for can now be perused. Oh, and if you live in Canada or Australia, let your member of Parliament know when you're approaching your ninetieth birthday. For Canadians, the governor general will honor the occasion with a greeting. For Australians, the prime minister will send a greeting. However, if you live in the United States or South Africa, tough.

Here's a caution. The flattering appraisals you attract from all sides may mislead you. "Oh, you're ninety and you can still . . ." Still what? Breathe? Talk? Walk? You can easily fall into the habit of boasting about your age, injecting the information into conversations for startling effect and possible compliments. The message this sends to the body is *Okay, I've made it. Now I can die peacefully.*

Don't Turn a Blind Eye to Life

Neighbors who have endured a heart attack walk past my home every day. But theirs isn't a joyful stroll. You can read sadness on their faces: they're engaging in an arduous, joyless task made necessary by illness. With eyes downcast, looking no more than a few yards ahead of them, they plod a lonely path in pursuit of longer life — while ignoring it! Their trek is a form of self-imposed punishment; they don't see the trees, flowers, birds, bees, and butterflies. What a pity! They might be wiser to walk on a treadmill, where at least they wouldn't have to be concerned about traffic (there are no sidewalks on our street).

And yet we might wonder whether they see any less of their environment than people who wear earphones, text messages, or make phone calls while walking. According to studies reported in the *New York Times*, these activities exact an insidious cost, inducing a hunched posture that promotes both physiological and psychological ailments. A stiff neck, yes, but lamentably a dwarfed mind as well.

It's hardly surprising that the concept of mindfulness has burst upon the scene. Failing to enjoy the immediate moment and the glory of one's surroundings has been found to lead to a rash of ailments: anxiety, depression, insomnia, stress, ADHD, substance abuse. Awaking to the present is therefore conducive to our health. Think about it. We can enjoy only the present moment. We can't live yesterday or tomorrow; we're stuck in the present, so we would be wise to accept the fact and enjoy it. If our surroundings are pleasant, we should alert ourselves to the fact, state it aloud in confirmation, and extract whatever treasure we can from the scene. If we look for magic in our environment, we increase our chances of finding it.

When I'm out with the dogs, I sometimes have to pull myself up sharply, glance around at the trees, and realize that the moment and the surroundings constitute the most important part of my entire day.

Speaking of noticing trees, with some caution I admit that I sometimes speak to them (they rarely respond), and as a member of Tree Huggers Anonymous (correction: being the only member probably makes me president), I even hug them occasionally.

(*Is it safe to be near this man? Well, no closer than the printed page.*) But then, I have an affection for trees, as I have for dogs. Perhaps it's a legacy of my early days, when I painted landscapes and admired those who depicted trees better than I could. In any case, hugging a tree releases body chemicals that make me feel good. And feeling good, of course, is an important contributor to staying healthy.

Imagination can by itself similarly cause the body to release one of its "feel-good" chemicals, which include endorphins, oxytocin, serotonin, and dopamine. The threat of danger, on the other hand, causes the body to release a surge of stress hormones, which include cortisol. Scientists have known for years that elevated cortisol levels increase risk for depression, mental illness, and shorter life expectancy. Continuing stress can interfere with learning and memory; can lower immune function and even bone density; and can increase weight gain, blood pressure, cholesterol, and heart disease. That's a killer combination. In fact, studies conducted at Johns Hopkins Hospital show that a feeling of intense fear can kill people; this includes children who have died on amusement park rides and car accident victims who actually sustained only minor physical injury.

Researchers at Carnegie Mellon University checked the stress levels and number of hugs received (or given) by 404 volunteers for two weeks. Their results, published in *Psychological Science*, showed that social support and frequent hugs protected people from infections caused by stress. Stressed people who received hugs regularly were roughly 60% less likely to get sick.

Of course, the studies were carried out with people-huggers. If you have someone handy to hug, good. Otherwise, there are plenty of trees available. I don't think it really matters so much what or whom you hug — a loved one, your dog, a tree — it's the feeling, the affection that you put into your hug that's important. The body's chemical reaction is the same in each case. So pick your tree, and remember — with feeling! Next patient, please.

Staying Healthy

Some readers may think that by the time they reach ninety, scientists will have found near-magical rejuvenating potions to guarantee health. We might hope so. Unfortunately, betting on a pill to secure deliverance from an unhealthy lifestyle is an unsound gamble. New "cures" are likely to suffer the same fate as earlier ones. Viruses are prompt to modify their method of attack and come up with new, indestructible versions of their former selves.

When a new drug is discovered, it's invariably misused in a futile effort to fight viruses instead of bacteria. In the process, the infective agent generates new forms of itself that are resistant to the drug. Such was the fate of streptomycin, tetracycline, and methicillin, and there is no reason to believe that any new wonder drug will survive similar misuse. The World Health Organization warned us in 2014: "A post-antibiotic era in which common infections and minor injuries can kill is a very real possibility for the 21st century."

You may recall that I began jogging again. Jogging presented an excellent way to increase my pulse rate in a matter of minutes. Such exercise is important for the heart, of course. The medically recommended upper limit for pulse rate varies with age. You can find yours by deducting your age from 220. For example, if you're forty-five years old, deduct 45 from 220 and you end up with 175. That's as high as your pulse should safely beat.

Now for the sad part. It dawned on me that, because of the half knee replacement in my left leg, I risked losing my ability to walk by continuing to jog, so I quit. But I found an alternative way to quickly boost my heart rate. I discovered a treadmill that provides varying degrees of incline. By setting it to its highest level of slant, I'm now able to get up to a puffing level of exertion quickly (at age ninety, that's 130 beats per minute). Of course, you can achieve a similar effect by running up and down the stairs in your house a few times.

Some Suggested Reading

This book deals with preventing illness, not curing it. However, some readers may suffer occasional (or even frequent) physical discomfort, and I'd be remiss not to mention a way to reduce perceived pain. The method is called "self-healing through imagery." Though the procedure sounds fanciful, even cloud-born, I ask anyone who is enduring physical distress to suspend judgment until they've studied the matter. What can you lose? What might you gain? My textbook is *Guided Imagery for Self-Healing* by Dr. Martin L. Rossman, though I'm sure others are available.

Before we part, I must express thanks to John Robbins, author of *Healthy at 100*, for all the information that has helped me appear knowledgeable. Similarly, to Joel Fuhrman, author of the books *Eat to Live* and *Super Immunity*, my gratitude. Readers can't do better than to read these works and learn more about matters on which I have briefly touched. Last, Dale Carnegie's *How to Win Friends and Influence People*, though eighty years old now, provides a mint of wisdom on dealing with others.

Depending on the content of the book and the way it's written, a nonfiction work often gives us access to the author's inner thoughts and character. I haven't found a more pleasant and admirable mind to enter than that of Jim Corbett, who stalked and killed man-eating tigers in India. Corbett constantly placed his life in danger to spare local villagers the threat of death in a most unpleasant form. His exploits are described in a simple, non-inflationary manner, almost as if anyone could do what he describes. Corbett was able to dispose himself comfortably on tree limbs to sleep at night when circumstances obliged (tigers can't climb trees). A marksman without equal, he was nevertheless quick to admit any error he made, and in doing so, set a refreshingly high mark for modesty. It's scant wonder I've read his book *Man-Eaters of Kumaon* several times.

I had completed writing this book when I became aware of *What Makes Olga Run?* This fascinating book uses ninety-year-old track star Olga Kotelko — holder of twenty-six world records — as a reference point to describe several ongoing studies being conducted of longevity-yielding practices. The book awakened me to the fact that I've been coddling myself — grooming a champion slacker — and compelled me to swing swiftly into a more taxing routine. The simple truth I learned is that each of us should occasionally push ourselves to our puffing, uncomfortable limit.

Is old age, then, a sort of battle? It is if you wish to maintain your tenancy on planet Earth. Old age provides a surprising continuum of physical burdens that you must either accept or counter. It's a tough war. *Growing Old Is Not for Sissies* is a regrettable truth. It's also the title of a book by Etta Clark, a coffee-table tome that should be on every coffee table. This publication contains large photos of older people — some in their nineties — who excel in various physical sports. Their prodigious achievements definitely snap one awake.

Many moons have passed since I began this opus. I'm now ninety-one (happy birthday to me!). Oh, and I'm not too sure I should mention this, but I've started talking to Fred. Not a peep out of him yet, but if he starts responding, I know the right people to call.

If you reach ninety and the content of this book has helped you achieve that age in a healthy and spirited manner, it has served its purpose.

Onward to one hundred.

Appendix

Here are some ideas to spark your imagination for the creative writing exercise in Chapter 6.

A Comedy

Early evening fog was moving in at the Wheaton crossing. No trains now until 05:45, when the Linden early-bird would roar through. Abez, the station master, yawned, tore April 16, 1945, from the desk calendar and flicked off the lights. In bed quickly, he hadn't been asleep more than an hour when his ears caught the sound of — What? Couldn't be! A train approaching. With clanging bell and hissing steam, a locomotive was screeching to a lazy halt. By the time Abez had donned pants and slippers, the engine had started up and was puffing slowly away. That's when he looked out to see . . . nothing. There was no train. Yet a lone figure stood on the wet, steaming platform holding a suitcase.

The apparition moved in a shuffling manner toward the depot and began mounting the steps to the elevated control room. Abez could now see that the figure was wearing a battered stovepipe hat, grubby clothes, and an immense scarf that trailed down over his feet and beyond. Abez grabbed a knife, his only weapon at hand, as the figure thumped violently on the door. Summoning all his courage, Abez swung the door open, knife ready at his side.

A deep, croaking voice with a British accent thundered, "Ebenezer Scrooge?"

"Huh? It's Abez Hawkins, mister. What do you want?"

The figure seemed stupefied by this news. "Well, where's Ebenezer, then?"

"Who's Ebenezer?" Then, with a gasp of understanding, Abez added, "Say, your name isn't Jacob Marley, is it?"

Looking stunned, the figure scratched a stubble of gray beard. "How did you know?"

"Well, I read *A Christmas Carol* a long time ago and —"

"There, then the secret's out. My cover's gone."

"Look, sweetie, you've warped into the wrong time period. You'll have to beat it. I've gotta get some sleep."

"I can't go. I used all my ectoplasmic power for the train effect."

Enough. There is now an opportunity to branch into all manner of comic entanglements. Here's a ghost imprisoned in the present time because he hasn't sufficient psychic power to return to his ethereal home. This slightly senile apparition, it turns out, has short-term memory loss and forgets how to work his dimmer switch (to become invisible or even semitransparent). And he's obliged to accompany Abez on his daily errands dressed in his odd other-century getup. Might this seed further ghoulish humor blossoms?

A Romance

Early evening fog was moving in at the Wheaton crossing. No trains now until 05:45, when the Linden early-bird would roar through. Abez, the station master, yawned, tore April 16, 1945, from the desk calendar and flicked off the lights. In bed quickly, he hadn't been asleep more than an hour when his ears caught the sound of — What? Couldn't be! A train approaching. With clanging bell and hissing steam, a locomotive was screeching to a lazy halt. By the time Abez had donned pants and slippers, the engine had started up and was puffing slowly away. That's when he looked out to see . . . nothing. There was no train. Yet a lone figure stood on the wet, steaming platform holding a suitcase.

Austen hit the Save button, then Print. Grabbing his hat, coat, and the hard copy he raced down three flights of stairs onto the darkened street. Dammit! Snowing. Buses running late. By the time he got to the university, class had started.

Snowdon, the instructor, beamed in mock pleasure. "Ah, Austen Scott! Thank you for coming. I think the demonic hazards that seemingly always prevent your punctual arrival might make an excellent future assignment for the class."

Austen felt his face flush as he made for his seat. Strangely, it was occupied by a new student. Realizing her error, she rose and moved elsewhere.

Later Snowdon made up for his earlier caustic criticism by commenting grandly on Austen's opening paragraph. "I think we have another Hemingway here. Someday we may measure our worth by the fact that we shared the company of one Austen Scott, uh, before the world discovered him."

Class ended. After receiving his classmates' congratulations, Austen rose and felt around the shelf under the desk for his things. He found an iPhone. At the same moment, the girl who had been occupying his seat at the beginning of class seemed to be frantically looking for something. She was attractive, with a capital A.

Austen held up the phone, and her face radiated relief.

"Uh, finders keepers, losers weepers, some say. But tell you what, if you'll join me for a coffee, I'll make you a gift of this rare object."

She smiled.

Well, they have coffee. She has a car and drives him home. He refuses to get out until she promises to have supper with him some night. Next thing they're in love, so now you "get your characters up a tree and throw rocks at them." Tear the two apart in a heart-wrenching manner that prevents any possible reunion. Then — *ta-da!* — let love find a way.

A Murder Mystery

Early evening fog was moving in at the Wheaton crossing. No trains now until 05:45, when the Linden early-bird would roar through. Abez, the station master, yawned, tore April 16, 1945, from the desk calendar and flicked off the lights. In bed quickly, he hadn't been asleep more than an hour when his ears caught the sound of — What? Couldn't be! A train approaching. With clanging bell and hissing steam, a locomotive was screeching to a lazy halt. By the time Abez had donned pants and slippers, the engine had started up and was puffing slowly away. That's when he looked out to see . . . nothing. There was no train. Yet a lone figure stood on the wet, steaming platform holding a suitcase.

Greta's voice trailed off. She glanced up from the page. Mendel could no longer hear her. He was asleep. Correction, Mendel was dead.

Greta checked his pulse. Then, using a napkin to maintain his fingerprints, she rinsed the glass free of poison in the kitchen, swirled fresh soda water around the inside, and placed it back on the table beside him.

There was no need to hurry to call the police, so she mixed herself a drink. She'd need steady nerves for the tears and agonized performance she'd have to give for the reporters and police soon to invade Mendel J. Grant's mansion.

Right, there you are. A murder, a murderer, and the method of death. We could now direct the story in any one of several directions. Who is the victim? Is he important? Why did Greta want him out of the way? And who is she, anyway — his wife, housekeeper, companion, daughter? You can now plant false clues that will keep the police running around in circles until that moment when the lady is nailed or commits suicide, is murdered, or dies accidentally. Lots of choices, aren't there?

Index

57656084R00092

Made in the USA
Charleston, SC
19 June 2016